AF450147

NSAIDs

Non-Steroidal Anti-Inflammatory Drugs

An Overview

NSAIDs

Non-Steroidal Anti-Inflammatory Drugs

An Overview

Swarnlata Saraf

Reader

Institute of Pharmacy,

Pt. Ravishankar Shukla University,

Raipur (C.G) - 492010.

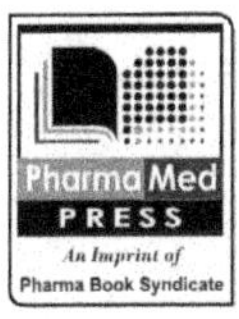

PharmaMed Press

An imprint of Pharma Book Syndicate

A Unit of BSP Books Pvt. Ltd.

4-4-309/316, Giriraj Lane,

Sultan Bazar, Hyderabad - 500 095.

Published by

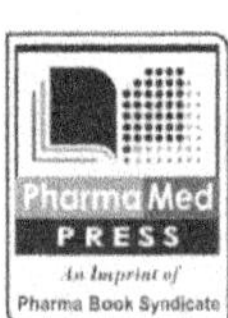

PharmaMed Press

An imprint of Pharma Book Syndicate

A unit of BSP Books Pvt. Ltd.

4-4-309/316, Giriraj Lane, Sultan Bazar, Hyderabad - 500 095.

Phone: 040-23445605, 23445688; Fax: 91+40-23445611

e-mail: info@pharmamedpress.com

ISBN : 978-93-5230-023-5 (HB)

Preface

It gives us immense pleasure in bringing out the first edition of the book NSAIDs: An Overview

Musculoskeletal disorders presents a serious socioeconomic burden that has and will continue to attract major research and development efforts aimed at elucidating the basis of the disease as well as developing effective new drug molecules as well as therapies. Non-steroidal anti-inflammatory drugs (NSAIDs) are the most frequently prescribed drugs worldwide in musculoskeletal disorders. These are categorized as 'over-the counter' (OTC) inavailability, and are also consumed on a non-prescription basis as well. The approach and purpose of this books are different from those of the several excellent books on the NSAIDs. No single book is available which covers all the different aspects of NSAIDs. Many drug molecules are available in the market but complete information on those molecules is not available in one book especially the recently invented molecules. Drug professionals, research scholars, graduate and undergraduate students of pharmacy all over the world face problems in knowing all about such molecules. We have made the efforts to compile information about NSAIDs at one place in this book. This book will be beneficial to all professionals working in hospitals, clinics, academia, nursing, drug stores, PG and research students of medicine and pharmacy.

The salient features of the book are

- It covers different areas of information viz; drug interactions, contraindications, warnings and combination of drugs
- FDA regulations for use of NSAIDs in clinics, hospitals and dispensaries to help in preparing and dispensing as well as nursing of NSAIDs.
- The physico-chemical properties with current literature review make this manuscript helpful to researcher of medical and pharmacy.
- The generic names of the drugs are given with brand names which are important and useful for physicians.

- Besides, all current information of individual drugs has been covered which make it useful in the drug information centre of different states as suggested by the WHO.

- Clinical aspects of NSAIDs

This book consists of 6 chapters.

Chapter I – Introduction, consists of general information of NSAIDs such as properties, classifications, brand names of drugs available all over the world, combinations, side effects, mechanism of action, warning and contraindications etc.

Chapter II, III, IV and V consist of specific physicochemical properties of individual drugs based on their chemical classification which covers interactions, clinical values and trade names etc.

Chapter VI consists of tabular information about individual drugs which is a ready reconer of NSAIDs.

There is no book for NSAIDs available in the market which has all information at one place; hence, this manuscript will cater the need of all interested professionals working in the field of NSAIDs.

We have tried to make this book as informative and exhaustive as possible within the constraints of time allotted to the subject in the curriculum of different universities. This book provides copious information about NSAIDs and points out their interactions and side effects.

We hope this book will be informative, beneficial and will fulfil the demands of the undergraduate and graduate students, budding researchers of the pharmacy, paramedical students as well as medical practitioners.

We are particularly indepted to our colleagues **Mr. Kamlesh Dashora** and **Mr. Gopal Garg** for their constant support to make this book.

-Author

Contents

Chapter 3

Enolic Acid Compounds

Chapter 4

Non Acidic Compounds

Chapter 5

Miscellaneous

Chapter 6

Tabular Information

Chapter 1

Introduction

Drugs from several diverse structural classes share anlgesic, antipyretic and anti-inflammatory activity. Nonsteroidal anti-inflammatory drugs (NSAIDs) use continues to expand at a remarkable rate due both to the broad spectrum of clinical applications for these medications and to the relatively recent introduction of the popular COX-2-selective inhibitors. The use of NSAIDs is particularly prevalent in patients with a variety of musculoskeletal conditions and injuries. Non-steroidal anti-inflammatory drugs (commonly called NSAIDs) reduce pain significantly in patients with arthritis, low back pain, and soft tissue pain. However, NSAIDs have important adverse effects, including gastrointestinal (GI) bleeding, peptic ulcer disease, hypertension, edema, and renal disease. More recently, some NSAIDs have also been associated with an increased risk of myocardial infarction.

NSAIDs reduce pain and inflammation by blocking *cyclo-oxygenases (COX)*, enzymes that are needed to produce *prostaglandins*. Most NSAIDs block two different cyclo-oxygenases, called COX-1 and COX2. COX-2, found in joint and muscle, contributes to pain and inflammation. NSAIDs cause bleeding because they also block the COX-1 enzyme, which protects the lining of the stomach from acid. NSAIDs differ in their selectivity for COX-2 how much they affect COX-2 relative to COX-1. An NSAID that blocks COX-2 but not COX-1 might reduce pain and inflammation in joints but leave the stomach lining alone.

In 1899, Bayer Corporation produced acetylsalicylic acid commercially for the first time. After this humble beginning more than 100 years ago, various other versions of nonsteroidal anti-inflammatory drugs (NSAIDs) have been introduced in the market. Today, NSAIDs are a commonly used class of medication found in numerous prescription and over-the-counter remedies. In many countries, they are one of the most frequently used types of medication, particularly for symptoms associated with osteoarthritis and other chronic musculoskeletal conditions. Their indications are far reaching, however, extending beyond simple bone, joint, and muscle pain. These indications include diverse medical conditions such as myofacial pain syndrome, gout, fever, dysmenorrhea, migraine headaches, the management of preoperative pain, and prophylaxis for stroke and myocardial infarction. With this broad spectrum of clinical applications, NSAID use continues to grow at a remarkable rate. Between 1984 and 1988, the number of patients receiving prescriptions for NSAIDs ballooned from 44 million to 70 million annually. In 1991, the worldwide market for NSAIDs was estimated to be $2 billion per year. By 1997, this number had increased to greater than $6 billion. These statistics emphasize the tremendous expansion in the use of NSAIDs, particularly in recent years. Specifically within the elderly population, the prevalence of NSAID use is even more remarkable. In a 1994 study out of Alberta, Canada, investigators discovered that 27% of elderly individuals received an NSAID prescription over the course of a 6-month time period. This broad use of NSAIDs in an elderly cohort at risk for metabolic bone disease and skeletal injury, coupled with the extensive use of NSAIDs in patients with bone and joint pathology, spawned research designed to examine the effects NSAIDs may impart on the process of bone healing. In fact, these investigations, carried out over the past several decades, produced some startling data. Numerous NSAIDs, including ibuprofen, indomethacin, aspirin, ketorolac, and naproxen, have all demonstrated inhibition of bone healing under various experimental conditions. More recently, examination of the new COX-2 inhibitors has yielded some important preliminary results as well. Although publicity has revolved around their link to increased cardiovascular events, data also support the notion that they also suppress bone formation and inhibit fracture healing.

Cyclooxygenase Enzyme (COX-1 and 2)

COX or prostaglandin H_2 synthatase (PGHS), first purified in 1976 and cloned in 1988, is a membrane of bound intracellular enzyme, which plays a key role in PG's synthesis from arachidonic acid. PG's are important mediators of many physiological processes; they regulate vascular homeostasis, kidney function, ovulation and parturition. These are also responsible for pain and fever, which accompanies inflammation and associated responses. The search for better drugs continued and researchers between 1989 and 1992 found that there were really two different COX enzymes. They are referred to as **"Cyclo-oxygenase-1 (COX-1) and Cyclo-oxygenase-2 (COX-2)"**. The genes for these two isoforms are located on separate chromosomes. Prostaglandins and thromboxanes generated via the COX-1 and COX-2 pathways are identical molecules and therefore have identical biological effects. Cyclooxygenase (COX), the key enzyme for synthesis of prostaglandins, exists in two isoforms (COX-1 and COX-2). COX-1 is constitutively expressed in the gastrointestinal tract in large quantities and has been suggested to maintain mucosal integrity through continuous generation of prostaglandins. COX-2 is induced predominantly during inflammation. On this premise selective COX-2 inhibitors not affecting COX-1 in the gastrointestinal tract mucosa have been developed as gastrointestinal sparing anti-inflammatory drugs. They appear to be well tolerated by experimental animals and humans following acute and chronic (three or more months) administration. However, there is increasing evidence that COX-2 has a greater physiological role than merely mediating pain and inflammation. Thus gastric and intestinal lesions do not develop when COX-1 is inhibited but only when the activity of both COX-1 and COX-2 is suppressed. Selective COX-2 inhibitors delay the healing of experimental gastric ulcers to the same extent as non-COX-2 specific non-steroidal anti-inflammatory drugs (NSAIDs). Moreover, when given chronically to experimental animals, they can activate experimental colitis and cause intestinal perforation. The direct involvement of COX-2 in ulcer healing has been supported by observations that expression of COX-2 mRNA and protein is up regulated at the ulcer margin in a temporal and spatial relation to enhanced epithelial cell proliferation and increased expression of growth factors. Moreover, there is increasing evidence that up regulation of COX-2 mRNA and protein occurs during exposure of the gastric mucosa to noxious agents or to ischaemia reperfusion. These observations support the concept that COX-2 represents (in addition to COX-1) a further line of defence for the gastrointestinal mucosa necessary for maintenance of mucosal integrity and ulcer healing.

Mechanism of Action of NSAIDs

Since the first production of acetylsalicylic acid by Felix Hoffman, investigations into the mechanism of action of NSAIDs have provided a better understanding of the manner in which these drugs achieve their effects. Specifically, NSAIDs have been found to interfere with the production of certain types of prostaglandins (PGs), a form of eicosanoid, which have a multitude of effects on blood vessels, nerve endings, and cells involved in the inflammatory cascade. Eicosanoid synthesis begins with the release of arachidonate from membrane phospholipids via the activity of phospholipase A_2 (PLA_2). Subsequently, two different cyclooxygenase (COX) isozymes convert arachidonic acid into various PGs. It is here that NSAIDs, by interfering with the activity of the COX enzymes, inhibit the production of PGs (Fig. 1.1)

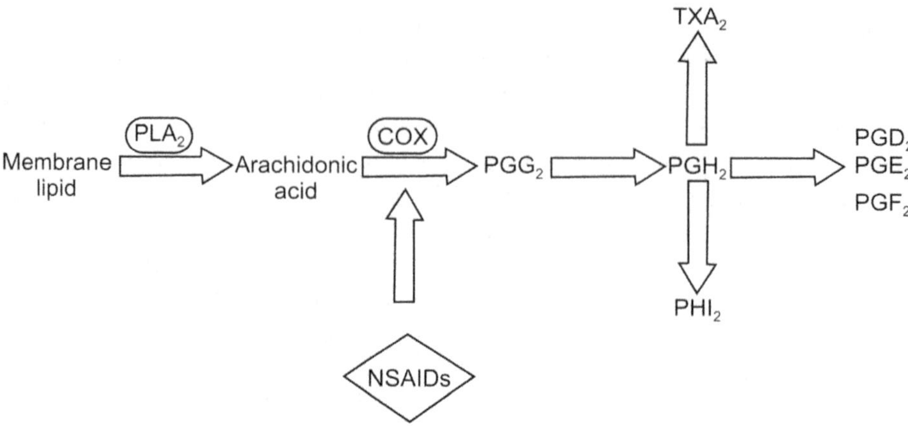

Fig. 1.1 Pathway for the generation of arachidonic acid metabolites and the site of the inhibitory activity of NSAIDs.

PGI_2 causes vasodilation and inhibits platelet aggregation, TXA_2 causes vasoconstriction and promotes platelet aggregation, and PGD_2, PGE_2, and PGF_2 cause vasodilation and potentiate edema. The production of PGG_2, PGH_2, PGI_2, PGD_2, PGE_2, PGF_2, and TXA_2 are all decreased by the inhibition of the COX enzymes by NSAIDs. PLA_2, phospholipase A_2; COX, cyclooxygenase; NSAIDs, nonsteroidal anti-inflammatory drugs; PGG_2, prostaglandin G_2; PGH_2, prostaglandin H_2; PGI_2, prostacyclin; PGD_2, prostaglandin D_2; PGE_2, prostaglandin E_2; PGF_2, prostaglandin F_2; TXA_2, thromboxane A_2.

Although closely related, the COX enzymes differ in certain important respects (Table 1.1). COX-1 serves as a constitutive enzyme located in a wide range of various tissue types such as the gastric mucosa, kidneys, and intestine. At these sites, it functions in the production of PGs necessary for normal cell activity but does not appear to play a role in the inflammatory process. Conversely, COX-2 is an inducible enzyme that operates as "an immediate early response gene product in inflammatory and immune cells." At sites of injury and inflammation, macrophages, fibroblasts, and synovial cells release COX-2, which subsequently upregulates the production of PGs involved in the inflammatory response. Classically, NSAIDs have inhibited the activity of COX-1 as much or more than COX-2. For instance, indomethacin and sulindac act primarily on COX-1 while meclofenamate and ibuprofen affect COX-1 and COX-2 equally. This activity results in the desired outcome of decreased inflammation via the inhibition of COX-2; however, it also serves to inhibit the PG production via COX-1, which is necessary for normal cell functioning such as cytoprotection in the stomach. Recently, drugs such as celecoxib and rofecoxib have been developed that target the COX-2 enzyme more specifically. Celecoxib, for example, demonstrates approximately 375 times more selectivity for COX-2 than for COX-1. These highly selective COX-2 inhibitors were created with the goal of interfering with the production of PGs manufactured via the COX-2 pathway, which are involved in inflammation while simultaneously sparing the PGs produced via COX-1 that are necessary for normal tissue function.

Table 1.1 Differences between COX-1 and COX-2 Enzymes.

	COX-1	COX-2
Expression	Constitutive	Inducible
Distribution	Wide and varied	Inflammatory and immune cells
Function	Normal cell activity	Inflammation
Inhibition	Traditional NSAIDs	New COX-2-specific NSAIDs

Selective COX-2 Inhibitors

Dexamethasone was the first pharmacological agent discovered that selectively blocks COX-2 induction. When cells are stimulated with cytokines, growth factors, or bacterial lipopolysaccharide endotoxin, the induced COX-2 expression observed is rapidly inhibited by dexamethasone. There are physiologic conditions, however, in which prostaglandin synthesis appears dependedent on constitutive COX activity, such as in the kidney or vasculature; under these circumstances, administration of glucocorticoids does not alter prostaglandin production *in-vivo*, suggesting a specific function for COX-1 in these tissues.

The effect of endogeneous glucocorticoids on the expression of the COX-2 enzyme, in both normal and diseased animals, was evaluated in animals rendered glucocorticoid deficient by adrenalectomy (ADX). Administration of endotoxin to these ADX animals further induced COX-2 expression, prostaglandin synthesis and increased mortality. Administration of glucocorticoids to the ADX animals inhibited COX-2 expression, decreased prostaglandin synthesis and protected animals from endotoxin induced death. Renal prostaglandin output was unchanged by adrenalectomy, administration of endotoxins or dexamethasone. These findings suggest that under normal physiologic conditions endogeneous glucocorticoids maintain a tonic inhibition of COX-2 expression. Depletion of glucocorticoids or the presence of an inflammatory stimulus such as endotoxins causes rapid induction of COX-2 enzyme resulting in an exacerbated inflammatory response.

Mechanistically, corticosteroids inhibit COX enzyme and prostaglandin production at the level of transcript expression or stability rather than a direct effect on enzyme activity. There are significant data, both *in–vitro* and *in-vivo*, that inhibition of COX-2 is an important mechanism by which steroids modulate inflammation. Unfortunately the wide array of pharmacologic actions observed after long term administration of glucocorticoids often results in serious side effects that limit their clinical utility, including fluid and electrolyte imbalance, decreased bone density, immunosuppression and Cushing like symptoms.

With the discovery of COX-2 and the increasing knowledge of its role in inflammation, the therapeutic advantage of a selective COX-2 inhibitor versus a traditional, nonselective NSAID became evident. Using expressed recombinant enzymes, it was reported that the current NSAIDs inhibit both COX-1 and COX-2. The various NSAIDs and COX-2 inhibitors differ in their relative inhibition of COX-1 and COX-2. The ability of a drug to inhibit a COX enzyme can be expressed as the IC_{50}, the concentration that inhibits 50 percent of prostanoid synthesis in the assay system. Calculation of a COX-2/COX-1 ratio (i.e., the ratio of the IC_{50} value for COX-2 divided by the IC_{50} value for 1) can provide a standard for comparing the selectivity of an NSAID for one or the other of the isoforms. NSAIDs that preferentially inhibit COX-2 relative to COX-1 have a COX-2/COX-1 activity ratio of less than 1. Comparision of these ratios among systems are limited by the variability in the assay conditions. Some of these differences reflect characterstics of the study agents, such as protein binding and lipohilicity that differentially affect the free drug concentration or the drug's ability to access the COX enzyme in each assay system, while others reflects the assay conditions themselves, such as the duration and temperature of incubation. Some of the differences may be related to the animal species from which the cells or COX enzyme for assay were taken, because COX enzymes are not completely conserved among mammals.

Classifications of NSAIDs

(A)   Chemical Classification

1. Carboxylic Acid

(i)   Salicylic acids and esters

Asprin, Diflunisal, Benorylate, Trisalicylate, Salsalate, Sodium salicylate

(ii) Acetic acid

Phenylacetic acids

Diclofenac, Aceclofenac, Fentiazac, Fenclofenac

Carbo and hetrocyclic acids

Etodolac, Indomethacin, Sulindac, Tolmetin, Tenidep, Zomepirac, Clopirac, Ketorolac, Tromethamine

(iii) Propionic acids

Carprofen, Fenbufen, Flurbiprofen, Ketoprofen, Oxaprozin, Suprofen, Tiaprofenic acid, Ibuprofen, Naproxen, Fenoprofen, Indoprofen, Benoxaprofen, Pirprofen

(iv) Fenamic acids

Flufenamic, Mefenamic, Meclofenamic, Niflumic

2. Enolic acids

Pyrazolones

Oxyphenbutazone, Phenylbutazone, Azapropazone, Feprazone

Oxicams

Piroxicam, Sudoxicam, Isoxicam, Tenoxicam, Meloxicam

3. Nonacidic compounds

Nabumetone, Proquazone, Fluproquazone,Tiaramide, Befexamac, Flunizole, Tinoridine

4. Miscellenaeous

Diaryl- substituted furanones

Rofecoxib

Diaryl-substituted pyrazoles

Celecoxib

Sulfonanilides

Nimesulide

(B)   Classification according to half lives

1. Nonsteroidal anti-inflammatory drugs with short half lives

(i)   Diclofenac

(ii)   Etodolac

    (iii)   Fenprofen

    (iv)   Flurbiprofen

    (v)   Ibuprofen

    (vi)   Indomethacin

    (vii)   Ketoprofen

    (viii)   Ketorolac

    (ix)   Tolmetin

    (x)   Meclofenamate

2. Nonsteroidal anti-inflammatory drugs with long half lives

    (i)   Diflunisal

    (ii)   Nabumetone

    (iii)   Naproxen

    (iv)   Oxaprozin

    (v)   Phenylbutazone

    (vi)   Piroxicam

    (vii)   Sulindac

(C)   Classification according to COX selectivity

1. Nonselective COX inhibitors

    (i)   Aspirin

    (ii)   Sodium salicylate

    (iii)   Salasalate

    (iv)   Diflunisal

    (v)   Indomethacin

    (vi)   Sulindac

    (vii)   Tolmetin

    (viii)   Diclofenac

    (ix)   Ketorolac

    (x)   Ibuprofen

    (xi)   Naproxen

    (xii)   Flurbiprofen

(xiii)   Ketoprofen

(xiv)   Fenoprofen

(xv)   Oxaprozin

(xvi)   Mefenamic acid

(xvii)   Meclofenamic acid

(xviii)   Piroxicam

(xix)   Meloxicam

(xx)   Nabumetone

2. Selective COX inhibitors

(i)   Rofecoxib

(ii)   Celecoxib

(iii)   Nimesulide

(iv)   Etodolate

(v)   Valdecoxib

Therapeutic Effects

All NSAIDs are antipyretic, analgesic, and anti-inflammatory, but there important differences in their activities. For example, acetaminophen is antipyretic and analgesic but is only weakly anti-inflammatory. The reasons for such differences are not fully understood, but differential sensitivity of enzymes in tissue environments may be important. When employed as analgesics, these drugs usually are effective only against pain of low-to-moderate intensity. Although their maximal effects are much lower, they lack the unwanted effects of the opioids on the central nervous system (CNS), including respiratory depression and the development of physical dependence. NSAIDs do not change the perception of sensory modalities other than pain. Chronic postoperative pain or pain arising from inflammation is particularly well controlled by NSAIDs, whereas pain arising from the hollow viscera is usually not relieved.

As antipyretics, NSAIDs reduce the body temperature in febrile states. Although all such drugs are antipyretics and analgesics, some are not suitable for either routine or prolonged use because of their toxicity; phenylbutazone is an example.

NSAIDs find their chief clinical application as anti-inflammatory agents in the treatment of musculoskeletal disorders, such as rheumatoid arthritis, osteoarthritis, and ankylosing spondylitis. In general, NSAIDs provide only symptomatic relief from the pain and inflammation associated with the disease and do not arrest the progression of pathological injury to tissue during severe episodes. Two other uses of NSAIDs that depend upon their capacity to block prostaglandin biosynthesis also deserve mention. Prostaglandins have been implicated in the maintenance of potency of the ductus arteriosus, and indomethacin and related agents have been used in neonates to close the ductus when it has remained patent. The release of prostaglandins by the endometrium during menstruation may be a cause of severe cramps and other symptoms of primary dysmenorrhea; treatment of this condition with NSAIDs has met with considerable success.

Analgesic Effects

Generally all of the NSAIDs relieve pain when used in doses relatively lower than those required to demonstrate supreession of inflammation. When employed as analgesics, these drugs usually are effective only against pain of low-to-moderate intensity, such as dental pain. The analgesic action of NSAIDs is generally considered to be peripheral as opposed to the central effect of narcotics. Chronic postoperative pain or pain arising from inflammation is particularly well controlled by NSAIDs, whereas pain arising from the hollow viscera usually is not relieved.

Antipyretic Effects

The NSAIDs, but not colchicines, effectively suppress fever in humans and experimental animals. It has been postulated that PGE_2 produced in the organism vasculosum laminae terminalis (OVLT) generates neuronal signals that activate the termoregulatory center in the preoptic area of the anterior hypothalamus, which is situated closed to OVLT. PGE_2 synthesis is stimulated by cytokines such as interleukin-1, which are released by the action of pyrogens such as LPS. Although the expression of COX-2 in the central nervous system is increased after LPS, the induction is not in neurons but in the endothelium of cranial blood vessels and in the microglia. PGE_2 involved in the febrile response derives from COX-2 induced in non-neuronal cells, probably endothelial cells of the blood vessels perfusing the hypothalamus. Although there is little evidence that any one pharmacologic clinical antipyretic effect is superior to another based on therapeutic ratio, aspirin remains the least expensive and most readily available.

Side Effects

In addition to sharing many therapeutic activities, NSAIDs share several unwanted side effects, the most common is a propensity to induce gastric or intestinal ulceration that can sometimes be accompanied by anemia from the resultant blood loss. Patients who use NSAIDs on a chronic basis have about three times greater relative risk for serious adverse gastrointestinal events compared to nonusers. NSAIDs vary considerably in their tendency to cause such erosions and ulcers. Gastric damage by these agents can be brought about by at least two distinct mechanisms. Although local irritation by orally administered drugs allows back diffusion of acid into the gastric mucosa and induces tissue damage, parenteral administration also can cause damage and bleeding, correlated with inhibition of the biosynthesis of gastric prostaglandins, especially PGI_2 and PGE_2, which serve as cytoprotective agents in the gastric mucosa. These eicosanoids inhibit acid secretion by the stomach, enhance mucosal blood flow, and promote the secretion of cytoprotective mucus in the intestine; inhibition of their synthesis may render the stomach more susceptible to damage. All of the NSAIDs discussed in this chapter, with the exception of p-aminophenol derivatives, have a tendency to cause gastrointestinal side effects, ranging from mild dyspepsia and heartburn to ulceration of the stomach or duodenum, sometimes with fatal results. Administration of the PGE_1 analog misoprostol along with NSAIDs may prove beneficial in the prevention of duodenal and gastric ulceration produced by these drugs. It also is possible that enhanced generation of lipoxygenase products contributes to ulcerogenicity in patients treated with NSAIDs and that there may be an association with *Helicobacter pylori* infection.

Injury to the gastrointestinal mucosa

For evaluation of the validity of new potentially less toxic NSAIDs it is mandatory to clearly understand the pathogenesis of NSAID induced ulceration (Fig. 1.2). Probably because of their suppression of prostaglandin synthesis, NSAIDs as a group tend to cause gastric irritation and to exacerbate peptic ulcers. Both aspirin and non-aspirin NSAIDs inhibit the COX pathway of prostaglandin synthesis. This represents the basis of anti-inflammatory action but is also responsible for the development of side effects in the gastrointestinal tract and kidney as well as inhibition of platelet aggregation. Inhibition of prostaglandin synthesis can exert injurious actions on the gastric and duodenal mucosa as it abrogates a number of prostaglandin dependent defense mechanisms. Inhibition of COX leads to a decrease in mucus and bicarbonate secretion, reduces mucosal blood flow, and causes vascular injury, leucocyte accumulation, and reduced cell turnover, all factors that contribute to the genesis of mucosal damage. Within this broad spectrum of events, the microvascular damage appears to play a central role. Prostaglandins of the E and I series are potent vasodilators that are continuously produced by the vascular endothelium. Inhibition of their synthesis by an NSAID leads to vasoconstriction. Furthermore, inhibition of prostaglandin formation results in a rapid and significant increase in the number of neutrophils adhering to the vascular endothelium in both gastric and mesenteric venules. Adherence is dependent on expression of the β_2 integrin (CD11/CD18) on neutrophils and intercellular adhesion molecule on the vascular endothelium. Neutrophil adherence in turn causes microvascular stasis and mucosal injury through ischaemia and release of oxygen derived free radicals and proteases. The severity of experimental NSAID gastropathy was markedly reduced in rats rendered neutropenic by pretreatment with antineutrophil serum or methotrexate. Recently, Wallace and colleagues provided evidence for an isoenzyme specific role of COX in the homeostasis of the gastrointestinal microcirculation. Thus in rats, the selective COX-1 inhibitor SC-560 decreased gastric mucosal blood flows without affecting leucocyte adherence to mesenteric venules. In contrast, the selective COX-2 inhibitor celecoxib markedly increased leucocyte adherence but did not reduce gastric mucosal blood flow. Only concurrent treatment with the COX-1 and COX-2 inhibitor damaged the gastric mucosa, suggesting that reduction of mucosal blood flow and increase in leucocyte adhesion have to occur simultaneously to interfere with mucosal defence. Inhibition of prostaglandin synthesis thus plays a key role in induction of mucosal injury but does not represent the only pathway by which NSAIDs can damage the gastrointestinal mucosa. NSAIDs can also induce local damage at the site of their contact with the gastrointestinal mucosa. Topical application of NSAIDs increases gastrointestinaln permeability allowing luminal aggressive factors access to the mucosa. Aspirin and most non-aspirin NSAIDs are weak organic acids. In the acidic milieu of the stomach, they are converted into more lipid soluble cells. There, at neutral pH, they are reionised and trapped within the cell causing local injury. Having entered gastric mucosal epithelial cells, NSAIDs uncouple mitochondrial oxidative phosphorylation. This effect is associated with changes in mitochondrial morphology and a decrease in intracellular ATP and therefore a reduced ability to regulate normal cellular functions such as maintenance of intracellular pH. This in turn causes loss of cytoskeletal control over tight junctions and increased mucosal permeability. The ability of NSAIDs to uncouple oxidative phosphorylation stems from the extreme lipid solubility and position of a carboxyl group that acts as a proton translator. A further mechanism involved in the topical irritant properties of NSAIDs is their ability to decrease the hydrophobicity of the mucus gel layer of the gastric mucosa. Lichtenberger *et al* have demonstrated that the surface of the stomach is hydrophobic and that this represents a defence mechanism which can be reduced by various pharmacological agents, including NSAIDs. NSAIDs can convert the mucus gel from a non-wettable to a wettable state and in experimental animals this effect has been shown to persist for several weeks or months after discontinuation of NSAID administration. Gastric mucosal lesions can also occur in a non-acidic milieu, such as following rectal application. With oral administration, gastric acid however appears to enhance NSAID induced damage. More extensive and deeper erosions occur at low pH and an elevation in gastric pH above 4 is necessary to prevent this acid related component. Prostaglandins do not represent a unique pathway to protect the gastric mucosa. Nitric oxide (NO) has the potential to counteract potentially noxious effects of inhibition of prostaglandin synthesis, such as reduced gastric mucosal blood flow and increased adherence of neutrophils to the vascular endothelium of the gastric microcirculation. No has well characterised inhibitory effects on neutrophil activation/adherence demonstrated in various tissues.

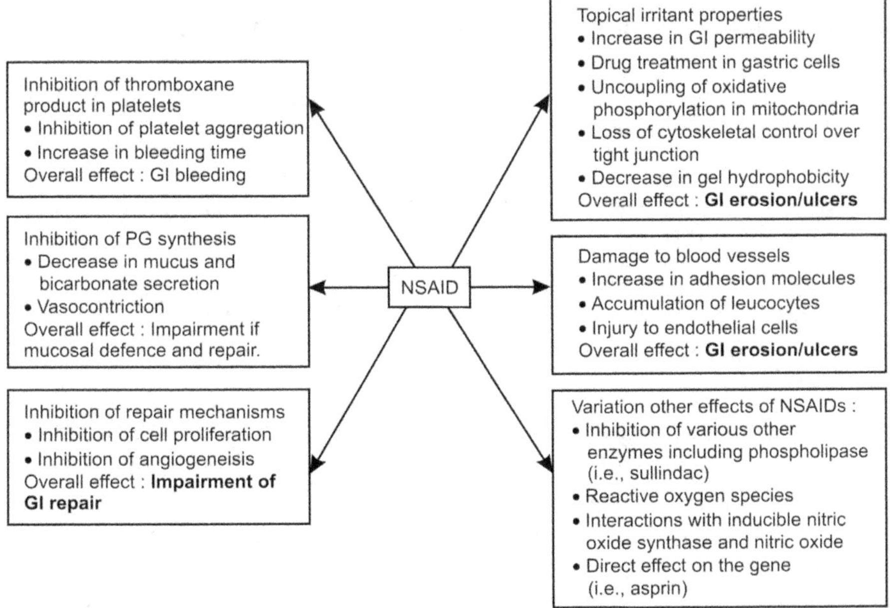

Fig. 1.2 Diagrammatic presentations of the mechanisms of non-steroidal anti-inflammatory drug (NSAID) injury to the gastrointestinal tract.

Other Effects

The other side effects of these drugs probably depend upon blockage of the synthesis of endogenous prostaglandins include disturbances in platelet function, the prolongation of gestation or spontaneous labor, and changes in renal function. Platelet function is disturbed because NSAIDs prevent the formation by the platelets of thromboxane A_2 (TXA$_2$), a potent aggregating agent. This accounts for the tendency of these drugs to increase the bleeding time. Aspirin is a particularly effective inhibitor of platelet function, because, as discussed above, the irreversible effects of aspirin on cyclooxygenase activity require new platelet production for restoration of enzyme activity. This "side effect" has been exploited in the prophylactic treatment of thromboembolic disorders. Prolongation of gestation by NSAIDs has been demonstrated in both experimental animals and women. Prostaglandins of the E and F series are potent uterotropic agents, and their biosynthesis by the uterus increases dramatically in the hours before parturition. It is thus hypothesized that prostaglandins have a major role in the initiation and progression of labor and delivery. Accordingly, some NSAIDs have been used as tocolytic agents to inhibit preterm labor.

NSAIDs have little effect on renal function in normal human subjects, presumably because the production of vasodilatory prostaglandins has only a minor role in sodium-replete individuals. However, these drugs decrease renal blood flow and the rate of glomerular filtration in patients with congestive heart failure, hepatic cirrhosis with ascites, chronic renal disease, or in those who are hypovolemic; acute renal failure may be precipitated under these circumstances. In individuals with these clinical conditions, renal perfusion is more dependent than in normal individuals upon prostaglandins that cause vasodilatation and thus oppose the increased vasoconstrictive influences of norepinephrine and angiotensin II that result from the activation of pressor reflexes.

In addition to their hemodynamic effects in the kidney, NSAIDs promote the retention of salt and water by reducing the prostaglandin-induced inhibition of both the reabsorption of chloride and the action of antidiuretic hormone. This may cause edema in some patients who are treated with NSAIDs; it also may reduce the effectiveness of antihypertensive regimens. These drugs promote hyperkalemia by several mechanisms, including enhanced reabsorption of K^+ as a result of decreased availability of Na^+ at distal tubular sites and suppression of the prostaglandin-induced secretion of renin. The latter effect may account in part for the usefulness of NSAIDs in the treatment of Bartter's syndrome, which is characterized by hypokalemia, hyperreninemia, hyperaldosteronism, juxtaglomerular hyperplasia, normotension, and resistance to the pressor effect of angiotensin II. Excessive production of renal prostaglandins may play an important part in the pathogenesis of this syndrome.

Although nephropathy is uncommonly associated with the long-term use of individual NSAIDs, the abuse of analgesic mixtures has been linked to the development of renal injury, including papillary necrosis and chronic interstitial nephritis. The injury often is insidious in onset, is usually manifest initially as reduced tubular function and concentrating ability, and may progress to irreversible renal insufficiency if misuse of analgesics continues. Females are involved more frequently than are males, and often there is a history of recurring urinary tract infection. Emotional disturbances are common, and other drugs may be abused concurrently. Despite numerous clinical observations and experimental studies in animals and human beings, insights concerning the mechanisms underlying NSAID-fostered renal injury are lacking. Phenacetin was suggested to be the nephrotoxic component of older analgesic mixtures (commonly, aspirin-phenacetin-caffeine, or "APC") and, therefore, was removed from these products. Although the incidence of analgesic nephropathy in some countries has subsequently declined, this has not been a universal result, especially in Australia. It is thus possible that chronic abuse of a variety of different NSAIDs or analgesic mixtures may cause renal injury in the susceptible individual. An acute interstitial nephritis also can occur as a rare complication of the use of NSAIDs.

Certain individuals display intolerance to aspirin and most NSAIDs; this is manifest by symptoms that range from vasomotor rhinitis with profuse watery secretions, angioneurotic edema, generalized urticaria, and bronchial asthma to laryngeal edema and bronchoconstriction, hypotension, and shock. Although rare in children, this syndrome may occur in 20% to 25% of middle-aged patients with asthma, nasal polyps, or chronic urticaria and can occur when these patients receive even small amounts (<80 mg) of aspirin. A subset of paitients with mastocytosis also may exhibit adverse reactions with the use of aspirin. Despite the resemblance to anaphylaxis, this reaction does not appear to be immunological in nature. Moreover, an individual who is intolerant to one NSAID may react when exposed to any of a variety of such agents, despite their chemical diversity, although nonacetylated salicylates appear less likely to produce these reactions than are aspirin and acetylated agents. Such patients also may react if they ingest tartrazine (FD&C Yellow No. 5 dye), which is found in many foods and beverages. The underlying mechanism for this hypersensitivity reaction to NSAIDs is not known, but a common factor appears to be the ability of the drugs to inhibit cyclooxygenase activity. This has prompted the hypothesis that the reaction reflects the diversion of arachidonic acid metabolism toward the formation of increased amounts of leukotrienes and other products of lipoxygenase pathways. This view is as yet unproven, and it does not explain why only a minority of patients with asthma or other predisposing conditions display the reaction. Even so, results in a small number of patients suggest that blockade of 5-lipooxygenase with the drug zileuton may prevent symptoms and signs of aspirin intolerance.

Drug Interactions

There are reciprocal influences between NSAID and other molecules in relation to absorption, to distribution and to elimination; in fact, eventhough the number of interaction is small, the clinical implications do seem to be important.

Actually different molecules exhibit a sort of gradient of intensity in relation to other molecules; the most outstanding aspects of these pharmacological interactions being a rearrangement of their relative dosages.

In any case the implications of these phenomena in regard to long-term treatment are not entirely clear.

Thus, while the interaction between NSAIDs and respectively alcohol, cimetidine, anticoagulant, antidiabetics, diuretics, B-adrenoreceptors is well known, the understding of long term concurrent administration of steroids, gold salts, penicillamine etc. is poor; this has been a very commonly encountered situations in rheumatology, not only in relation to the problem of toxicity, but also in relation to to possible reciprocal enhancement.

A further aspect of the problem lies in the tendency of many doctors to prescribe appropriate combinations of NSAIDs, whose usefulness and significance remains controversial. In fact the mere knowledge of their relative half life can not be considered a good enough basis on which to justify their indiscriminate use. In fact phenylbutazone inhibits the metabolism of warfarin, and therefore potentiates the anticoagulant effect of warfarin. Salicylates too affect the synthesis of of factor VII, IX and X. Similarly other NSAIDs do not seem to alter significantly the major parameters of coagulation especially prothrombin time: indomethacin, ibuprofen, naproxen, sulindac, diclofenac, indoprofen, piroxicam.

The NSAIDs least likely to interact with oral hypoglycemic agents are diclofenac, etodolac, fenoprofen, flurbiprofen, ibuprofen, indomethacin, ketoprofen, ketorolac, meclofenamate, tolmetin and sulindac. For the most part, NSAIDs do not affect the diuretic response to thiazides. Reversible acute renal failure and hyperkalemia may occur when indomethacin and triamterene are combined. Ethanol potentiates the gastrointestinal toxicity of NSAIDs.

Table 1.2 Provides a few potential interaction involving NSAIDs.

Pertubed Drugs	Pertubing Drug	Interaction Effect
Salicylate	Antacids	Increased rate of excretion with decreased salicylate levels
Anticoagulants	Phenylbutazone, oxyphenbutazone	Prolongation of prothrombin time due to inhibition of catabolism
Beta-blocker	All PG inhibiting NSAIDs	Blunting of hypotensive effect but not of negative chronotropic or intotropic effect.
Urinary alkalisers, antacids, corticosteroids	Aspirin	PABA may increase serum level. May potentiate the effects of anticoagulants, hypoglycemics, methotrexate. May antagonize uricosurics, spironolactone and tetracyclines
Celecoxib	Aspirin	May increase the occurance of stomach and intestinal ulcers
Rifampicin, methotrexate,warfarin and ACE inhibitors	Rofecoxib	-
Aspirin	Ibuprofen	Aspirin displaces ibuprofen from serum binding sites
Anticoagulants	Naproxen and ketoprofen	Enhances effect of oral anticoagulants, phenytoin, methotrexate, sulphonamides.
Salicylate	Glucocorticoids	Increased salicylate metabolism resulting in lowered plasma salicylate level.
Lithium	Many NSAIDs	Incrased plasma lithium level
Digoxin	Aspirin, many NSAIDs	May increase digoxin level
Piroxicam	Cimetidine	Increased plasma and half life of piroxicam
Hydralazine, prazosin	All PG inhibiting NSAIDs	Loss of hypotensive effects

NSAIDs in Varying Clinical Situations

The choice of an agent as an antipyretic or analgesic is seldom a problem. It is in the field of rheumatology that the decision becomes complex. The choice among NSAIDs for the treatment of arthritis is largely empirical. A drug may be chosen and given for a week or more; if the therapeutic effect is adequate, treatment should be continued unless toxicity occurs. Large variations are possible in the response of individuals to different NSAIDs, even when the drugs are structurally similar members of the same chemical family. Thus, a patient may do well on one propionic acid derivative (such as ibuprofen) but not on another. Initially, fairly low doses of the agent chosen should be prescribed to determine the patient's reaction. When the patient has problems sleeping because of pain or morning stiffness, a larger single dose of the drug may be given at night. A week is generally long enough to determine the effect of a given drug. If the drug is effective, treatment should be continued, reducing the dose if possible and stopping it altogether if it is no longer necessary. Side effects usually appear in the first weeks of therapy, although gastrointestinal ulceration may develop at later times. If the patient does not achieve therapeutic benefit from one NSAID, another compound should be tried, since, as noted above, there is a marked variation in the response of individuals to different but closely related drugs.

For mild arthropathies, the scheme outlined above, together with rest and physical therapy, probably will be effective. However, patients with a more debilitating disease may not respond adequately. In such cases, more aggressive therapy should be initiated with aspirin or another agent. It is best to avoid continuous combination therapy with more than one NSAID; there is little evidence of extra benefit to the patient, and the incidence of side effects generally is additive.

The choice of drugs for children is considerably restricted, and only drugs that have been extensively tested in children should be used. This commonly means that only aspirin, naproxen, or tolmetin should be prescribed. However, the association of Reye's syndrome in children with the administration of aspirin for the treatment of febrile viral illnesses precludes its use in this setting.

The use of any of the NSAIDs in pregnant women generally is not recommended. If such a drug must be given to a pregnant woman, low doses of aspirin are probably the safest. Although toxic doses of salicylates cause teratogenic effects in animals, there is no evidence to suggest that salicylates in moderate doses have teratogenic effects on the human fetus. In any case, aspirin should be discontinued prior to the anticipated time of parturition to avoid complications such as prolongation of labor, increased risk of postpartum hemorrhage, and intrauterine closure of the ductus arteriosus.

Many NSAIDs bind firmly to plasma proteins and thus may displace certain other drugs from the binding sites. Such interactions can occur in patients given salicylates or phenylbutazone together with warfarin, sulfonyl-urea hypoglycemic agents, or methotrexate; the dosage of such agents may require adjustment, or concurrent administration should be avoided. The problem with warfarin is accentuated because almost all NSAIDs disturb normal platelet function. Numerous other drug interactions are observed with NSAIDs.

A final important consideration in the selection of an NSAID for a patient is the cost of therapy, particularly since these agents frequently are used on a long-term basis. Generally speaking, aspirin is very inexpensive; ibuprofen is less expensive than indomethacin, and the cost of the newer drugs can be very high.

Marketed Dosage Form

These drugs are available in nearly every form:

- For oral administration they come in tablets, capsules or medicines. This is the most widely used form.

- Some NSAIDs are available as *injections*. This form is used for pain after surgical operations and also is very effective for the treatment of pain produced by kidney stones (renal colic).

- *Suppositories* are available. These are often used for post-operative pain and sometimes in chronic pain when the patient is unable to take medication by mouth.

- Creams, gels and foams to apply to the skin. These are not felt to be as effective, but some people do get considerable relief from their use.

Although non-oral routes of administration avoid the direct irritation of the stomach, they do not avoid the indigestion and ulcer risks, as these are caused by the chemical once it is in the blood stream. There are several formulations available in the market containing non-steroidal anti-inflammatory drugs with antipyretic or skeletal muscle relaxants (Table 1.3)

Table 1.3 Non steroidal anti-inflammatory combinations available in market.

S.No.	Type of combinations	actions	actions	indications	Dose
1.	**Ibuprofen** Ibuprofen S.R. 600 mg Ibuprofen 400 mg + paracetamol 500mg Ibuprofen 400 mg + paracetamol 325 mg Ibuprofen 400 mg + paracetamol 650 mg Ibuprofen 400 mg + paracetamol 500 mg + magnesium trisilicate 50 mg Ibuprofen 400 mg + paracetamol 500 + caffeine 65 mg Ibuprofen 200 mg + paracetamol 500 mg Ibuprofen 400 mg + paracetamol 333 mg	Analgesic effect: 30 Min. Anti-inflammatory effect: 7 days	4-6 hrs	Rheumatoid arthritis, ankylosing spondiltis, cervical spondiltis, primary dysmenorrhoea	400 mg t.i.d. S.R. preparation: b.i.d.
2.	**Flurbiprofen** Flurbiprofen100 mg Flurbiprofen 200 mg (S.R)	30-60 min	8-12 hrs.	Rheumatoid arthritis, ankylosing spondiltis, cervical spondiltis, primary dysmenorrhoea Post opera tive analgesia	50-100 mg. t.i.d S.R.: Once -daily

3.	**Ketoprofen** Ketoprofen 50 mg + Analgin 50 mg	30 min	6-8 hrs	Rheumatoid arthritis, gout, capsulitis of shoulder, primary dysm—enorrhoea, analgesia	100-150 mg in div. doses, Max: 300 mg daily
4.	**Naproxen** Naproxen 250 mg Naproxen 500 mg Naproxen 750 mg (S.R.): Daily	Analgesic effect: 30 Min. Anti-rheumatic effect: 2 weeks	7 hrs.	Rheumatoid arthritis, ankylosing spondiltis, cervical spondiltis, primary dysmenorrhoea acute gout, pelvic inflammation, tooth extraction, tendonitis, bursitis, juvenile arthritis	200 mg b.i.d. Gout: 700 mg Initially then 250 mg 8 hourly
5.	**Mefenamic acid** Mefenamic acid 250 mg+ Acetaminophen 500 mg Mefenamic acid 500 mg +acetaminophen 450 mg	1-2 hrs.	6 hrs.	Rheumatoid arthritis, ankylosing spondiltis, cervical spondiltis, primary dysmenorrhoea post operative analgesia	200-500 mg t.i.d.

S.No.	Type of combinations	Onset of actions	Duration of actions	Indications	Dose
6.	**Phenyl butazone** Phenyl butazone 125 mg + Propylphenazone 125 mg + Acetaminophen 250 mg	Analgesic effect: 2 hrs. Anti-rheumatic effect: 3-4 days.	Some effect last for 3-4 days	Rheumatoid arthritis, ankylosing spondiltis, rheumatic fever, osteoarthritis, after blunt injuries, fractures, tooth extraction, vasectomy, acute gout.	200mg t.i.d.
7.	**Oxyphenbutazone**	1-2 hrs.	Some effect last for 2 days	Rheumatoid disorder, inflammation	100 mg t.i.d
8.	**Indomethacin** Indomethacin 75 mg(S.R.) Indomethacin 25mg+paracetamol 325 mg	Analgesic effect: 30 min. Anti-rheumatic effect: 4-6hrs.	4-6 hrs.	Rheumatoid arthritis, ankylosing spondiltis. gout.	25-50 mg. t.i.d. 75-100 mg daily (S.R.)

Table 1.3 Contd…

S.No.	Type of combinations	Onset of actions	Duration of actions	Indications	Dose
9.	**Diclofenac** Diclofenac sod. 100 mg (S.R.) Diclofenac sod. 50 mg +seratiopeptidase 10 mg. Diclofenac pot. 50 mg +seratiopeptidase 10 mg Diclofenac sod. 50 mg +seratiopeptidase 10 mg +paracetamol 325 mg. Diclofenac sod. 50 mg +paracetamol 500 mg.	Analgesic effect: 1 hrs. Anti-rheumatic effect: 2 weeks.	Up to 12 hrs. Up to 24 hrs. (S.R.)	Rheumatoid arthritis, ankylosing spondiltis, cervical spondiltis, primary dysmenorrhoea post operative analgesia	100-500 mg daily: In divided dose
10.	**Piroxicam** Piroxicam-beta cyclodextrin 20 mg	Analgesic effect: 1 hrs. Anti-rheumatic effect: 7-12 days.	48-72 hrs	Rheumatoid arthritis, ankylosing spondiltis, cervical spondiltis, primary dysmenorrhoea post operative analgesia	20 mg daily In gout: 40 mg daily Post operative analgesia: 40 mg

Warnings

NSAIDs cannot be used (are contraindicated) in the following cases:

- Allergy to aspirin or any NSAIDs
- Aspirin should not be used under the age of 16 years
- During pregnancy
- During breast feeding
- On blood thinning agents (anticoagulants)
- Suffering from a defect of the blood clotting system (coagulation)
- Active peptic ulcer
- Care is needed if you have: asthma, kidney impairment, heart impairment, liver impairment

Symptoms of NSAIDs Overdose

Symptoms of overdose can be similar to the medication's side effects, but are usually more severe. Patients exhibiting any of these symptoms should contact their physicians immediately:

- Bluish color to fingernails, lips or skin
- Severe and lingering headache
- Nausea or vomiting
- Difficulty breathing
- Fast or pounding heartbeat
- Confusion, agitation or incoherence
- Blurred vision
- Skin rash
- Abdominal pain or diarrhea
- Convulsions or seizures
- Hemorrhage (heavy bleeding) from stomach or intestine

In rare cases, the patient may also go into a coma (prolonged unconsciousness).

FDA Medication Guidelines

All prescription medications have benefits and risks, but the risk of taking some medications are potentially greater than others for some patients. For the medications that have a "risk profile" that is greater than average, in some cases, the FDA has required the dispensing of a FDA approved "Medication Guide." In theory, these consumer-oriented-Medication Guides are supposed to help inform patients about specific adverse events that may occur from taking these medications. After reading a Medication Guide, patients should be able to better determine whether to take the medication or how to identify potentially serious adverse effects.

With each prescription for a medication with an FDA-approved Medication Guide, pharmacists should provide a copy of the Medication Guide. While pharmacists continue to be eager to provide patients with information on their medications, the implementation of the current FDA mandated program has made it more difficult for community retail pharmacies to provide Medication Guide information to consumers efficiently. In addition, many patients that receive Medication Guides may not find the information useful given the risk-focused nature of the communication, as well as the quantity of other written information that pharmacies are also voluntarily providing to their patients with their prescriptions.

The purpose of this guideline is to provide policy makers with an overview of the current status of the medication guide program and offer suggestions on how the communication of risk information to patients can be done more efficiently and effectively.

Distribution Programs

The Medication Guides for NSAIDs classes represent the majority of medication guides dispensed in community pharmacies. To facilitate distribution of these guides to community retail pharmacies, brand and generic manufacturers of these medications formed coalitions with the intention of providing pharmacies with a uniform version of medication guides which can be dispensed with any medication within that class.

Status

With encouragement by the FDA and the pharmacy community, manufacturers of NSAIDs have formed a coalition similar to that of the antidepressants and have created a uniform version of the NSAID medication guide which could be distributed to all patients receiving any NSAID. This coalition has distributed an initial shipment of hard-copy tear-off pads of NSAID Medication guides to pharmacies in the first week of April, 2006. Similar to the antidepressants, within the tear-off pads of medication guides, there is a re-order form to obtain more Medication Guides. This NSAID Medication Guide replenishment program is currently still available for pharmacies.

Guidelines

1. What is the most important information I should know about medicines called Non-Steroidal Anti-Inflammatory Drugs (NSAIDs)?

   NSAID medicines may increase the chance of a heart attack or stroke that can lead to death. This chance increases:

   • with longer use of NSAID medicines

   • in people who have heart disease

   NSAID medicines should never be used right before or after a heart surgery called a "coronary artery bypass graft (CABG)."

   NSAID medicines can cause ulcers and bleeding in the stomach and intestines at any time during treatment. Ulcers and bleeding:

   • can happen without warning symptoms

   • may cause death

The chance of a person getting an ulcer or bleeding increases with:

   • taking medicines called "corticosteroids" and "anticoagulants"

   • longer use

   • smoking

   • drinking alcohol

   • older age

   • having poor health

NSAID medicines should only be used:

   • exactly as prescribed

   • at the lowest dose possible for your treatment

   • for the shortest time needed

Possible side effects of Non-Steroidal Anti-Inflammatory Drugs (NSAIDs).

Serious side effects include:	Other side effects include:
• heart attack	• stomach pain
• stroke	• constipation
• high blood pressure	• diarrhea
• heart failure from body swelling (fluid retention)	• gas
• kidney problems including kidney failure	• heartburn
• bleeding and ulcers in the stomach and intestine	• nausea
• low red blood cells (anemia)	• vomiting
• life-threatening skin reactions	• dizziness
• life-threatening allergic reactions	
• liver problems including liver failure	
• asthma attacks in people who have asthma	

Get emergency help right away if you have any of the following symptoms:

- shortness of breath or trouble breathing
- chest pain
- weakness in one part or side of your body
- slurred speech
- swelling of the face or throat

Stop your NSAID medicine and call your healthcare provider right away if you have any of the following symptoms:

- nausea
- more tired or weaker than usual
- itching
- your skin or eyes look yellow
- stomach pain
- flu-like symptoms
- vomit blood
- there is blood in your bowel movement or it is black and sticky like tar
- unusual weight gain
- skin rash or blisters with fever
- swelling of the arms and legs, hands and feet

These are not all the side effects with NSAID medicines. Talk to your healthcare provider or pharmacist for more information about NSAID medicines.

Other Information

- Aspirin is an NSAID medicine but it does not increase the chance of a heart attack. Aspirin can cause bleeding in the brain, stomach, and intestines. Aspirin can also cause ulcers in the stomach and intestines.

- Some of these NSAID medicines are sold in lower doses without a prescription (over –the –counter). Talk to your healthcare provider before using over –the –counter NSAIDs for more than 10 days.

Prescription NSAID

Generic Name	Tradename
Celecoxib	Celebrex
Diclofenac	Cataflam, Voltaren, Arthrotec (combined with misoprostol)
Diflunisal	Dolobid
Etodolac	Lodine, Lodine XL
Fenoprofen	Nalfon, Nalfon 200
Flurbirofen	Ansaid
Ibuprofen	Motrin, Tab-Profen, Vicoprofen (combined with hydrocodone), Combunox (combined with oxycodone)
Indomethacin	Indocin, Indocin SR, Indo-Lemmon, Indomethagan
Ketoprofen	Oruvail
Ketorolac	Toradol
Mefenamic Acid	Ponstel
Meloxicam	Mobic
Nabumetone	Relafen
Naproxen	Naprosyn, Anaprox, Anaprox DS, EC-Naproxyn, Naprelan, Naprapac (copackaged with lansoprazole)
Oxaprozin	Daypro
Piroxicam	Feldene
Sulindac	Clinoril
Tolmetin	Tolectin, Tolectin DS, Tolectin 600

Drug Information for Pharmacist:

Pharmacists have a responsibility to provide sufficient information and counseling to enable patients and / or their caretakers to achieve informed and judicious use of NSAIDs. The Table 1.4 provides suuficint informations to the pharmacists for the patient counseling and dispensing of NSAIDs.

Table 1.4 NSAIDs drug information for Pharmacists.

Drug	Clinical applications	Cautionary instructions	Dosing in relation to food	Side Effects	
				Common/Mild	Rare/serious
Aceclofenac Drugs Contraindicated: NA	Traetment of dental pain, postoperative pain, rheumatoid	Caution in case of previous history of gastrointestinal ulceration, bleeding, or perforation, renal dysfunction, hypertension or cardiac conditions aggravated by fluid retention and edema, history of liver dysfunction, preexisting infection, History of coagulation defects	N/A	Gastric discomfort or gastralgia mild, nausea, heartburn, erythema and itching	Leukocytoclastic vasculitis and hemoptysis
Aspirin Drugs contraindicated: Avoid if hypersensitivity to other NSAIDs	Treatment of angina pectoris, chronic stable and unstable coronary artery bypass graft (CABG), percutaneous transluminal coronary angioplasty, carotid endarterctomy, fever, ischemic stroke, transient ischemia, myocardial infaraction treatment and prophylaxis pain, rheumatoid arthritis, juvenile rheumatoid arthritis, spondylo arthropathy, osteoarthritis, arthritis.	Cautions in case of pregnancy, breastfeecing, kidney problems or a history of ulcers, asthma. Advise to avoid alcohol. (Avoid alcohol within 12 hours of this medicine)	Advise to take with food	Dyspepsia, nausea and vomiting	Bleeding, gastrointestinal ulcers, Reye's syndrome, tinnitus, angioedema, bronchospasm.

Table 1.4 *Contd…*

Drug	Clinical applications	Cautionary instructions	Dosing in relation to food	Side Effects	
				Common/Mild	**Rare/serious**
Diclofenac **Drugs** **contraindicated** Avoid if hypersensitivity to aspirin or NSAIDs	Treatment of ankylosing spondylitis (delayed release tablets only), cataract removal, treatment of postoperative inflammation (ophthalmic product), corneal referactive surgery, relief of pain and photophobia (ophthalmic product), osteoarthritis, rheumatoid arthritis	Advise not to take aspirin while being treated with this medicine unless advised by doctor. This medicine may affect mental alertness and or co-ordination. Advise the patient that if affected, not to drive a motor vehicle or operate machinery.	Advise to take with food	Abdominal pain, rash, constipation, diarrhea, dyspepsia, flatulence, nausea, pruritus, dizziness, headache, tinnitus, edema, liver function test elevations, burning elevated ocular pressure, lacrimation, stinging (ophthalmic solutions), blurred vision, conjunctivitis, corneal deposits, corneal edema (ophthalmic solutions), corneal opacity, corneal lesions, ocular discharge, iritis(ophthalmic solutions)	GI ulceration, GI perforation, melena, vomiting, anemia, pancreatitis, jaundice, hepatitis, hepatic necrosis (rare), cirrhosis (rare), leucopenia, anaphylaxis (rare), hypertension, CHF, thrombocytopenia, purpura, aplastic anemia, hemolytic anemia (rare), agranulocytosis(rar), Aseptic meningitis(rare), seizures(rare), angioedema, erythema multiforme (rare), Stevens-Johnson syndrome (rare), protenuria, acute renal failure(rare), intestinal nephritis (rare), nephritic syndrome (rare), blurred vision, hearing loss (1-3%)

Drug	Clinical applications	Cautionary instructions	Dosing in relation to food	Side Effects	
				Common/Mild	**Rare/serious**
Etoricoxib\ Drugs Contraindicated: N/A	Treatment of osteoarthritis and rheumatoid arthritis	Caution in case of peptic ulcers, bleeding, liver and renal disorders	Advise to takeafter food	Headache, dizziness, fatigue, insomnia, nausea, vomiting, diarrhea, heart burn, taste disturbances, decreased appetite and flatulence	N/A
	Treatment of fever, self-medication of juvenile rheumatoid arthritis, osteoarthritis, pain, mild to moderate pain, self-medication of minor primary dysmenorrhea, rheumatoid arthritis.	Advise not to take aspirin while being treated with this medicine unless advised by doctor. This medicine may affect mental alertness and or co-ordination. Advise the patient that if affected, not to drive a motor vehicle or operate machinery.	Advise to take with food	Abdominal pain, rash, constipation, diarrhea, dyspepsia, flatulence, nausea, pruritus, dizziness, headache, tinnitus, edema, heart burn	Liver function test abnormalities, hepatitis, jaundice, GI bleeding, GI perforation, melena, pancreatitis, acute renal failure, azote-mia, hematuria, agranulocytosis, anemia, thrombo-cytopenia,neutropenia, hypertension, CHF, anaphylaxis, depression, insomnia, confusion, aseptic meningitis (rare), erythemea, mutiforme, Stevens-Johnson syndrome, hearing loss, amblyopia

Table 1.4 Contd...

Drug	Clinical applications	Cautionary instructions	Dosing in relation to food	Side Effects	
				Common/Mild	Rare/serious
Indomethacin **Drugs Contraindicated:** N/A	Treatment of acute gouty arthritis, acute painful shoulder: brursitis and tendonitis, ankylosing spondylitis, rheumatoid arthritis, osteoarthritis.	Advise not to take aspirin while being treated with this medicine unless advised by doctor. This medicine may affect mental alertness and or co-ordination. Advise the patient that if affected, not to drive a motor vehicle or operate machinery.	Advise to take with food	Abdominal pain, constipation, diarrhea, dyspepsia, flatulence, nausea, pruritus, dizziness, headache, tinnitus, edema, depression, somnolence, rectal irritation, tenesmus.	anaphylaxis, asthma, edema, pulmonary edema, GI bleeding, GI perforation, arrhythmias, CHF, chest pain, hypertension, agranulocytosis, anemia, jaundice, rash, leucopenia, thrombocytopenic purpura, asthma, hepatitis, Stevens-Johnson syndrome, toxic epidermal necrolysis, hematuria, intestinal nephritis, nephritic syndrome, renal failure, pulmonary hypertension, hyponatremia, hyperkalemia, aggravation of epilepsy or parkinsonism, convulsion, peripheral neuropathy, psychic disturbances, corneal deposits, deafness.

Table 1.4 *Contd...*

Drug	Clinical applications	Cautionary instructions	Dosing in relation to food	Side Effects	
				Common/Mild	Rare/serious
Ketoprofen **Drugs Contraindicated:** N/A	Treatment of fever, self-medication of osteoarthritis, pain, mild to moderate pain, self-medication of minor primary dysmenorrhea, rheumatoid arthritis.	Advise not to take aspirin while being treated with this medicine unless advised by doctor. This medicine may affect mental alertness and or co-ordination. Advise the patient that if affected, not to drive a motor vehicle or operate machinery.	Advise to take with food	Abdominal pain, rash, constipation, diarrhea, dyspepsia, flatulence, nausea, dizziness.	Impairment of renal function, renal failure, CHF, intestinal nephritis, allergic reaction, anaphylaxis, hypertension, melania, GI bleeding, GI perforation, liver function test abnormalities, agranulocytosis, hepatitis, jaundice, anemia, thrombocytopenia.
Piroxicam **Drugs Contraindicated:** N/A	Tratment of osteoarthritis, rheumatoid arthritis.	Advise not to take aspirin while being treated with this medicine unless advised by doctor. This medicine may affect mental alertness and or co-rdination. Advise the patient that if affected, not to drive a motor vehicle or operate machinery.	Advise to take with food, milk ir antacids to avoid stomach upset	Abdominal pain, rash, constipation, diarrhea, dyspepsia, flatulence, nausea, dizziness, headache, tinnitus, edema, heart burn, edema	anemia, Liver function test abnormalities, hepatitis, jaundice, GI bleeding, GI perforation, melena, thrombocytopenia, arrhythmias (rare) , CHF, hypertension, tachycardia, vasculitis (rare), intertstitial nephritis, nephritic syndrome, renal failure, anaphylaxis, multiforme, Stevens-Johnson syndrome (rare),

Table 1.4 *Contd…*

Drug	Clinical applications	Cautionary instructions	Dosing in relation to food	Side Effects	
				Common/Mild	Rare/serious
Celecoxib **Drugs** **Contraindicated:** **Sulfonamides**	Treatment of acute pain, familial adenomatous polyposis, osteoarthritis, primary dysmenorrhea, rheumatoid arthritis.	Caution should be exercised in ulcer patients	Advise to take with or without food.	Abdominal pain, diarrhea, dyspepsia, flatulence, nausea, dizziness, headache, back pain, edema, insomnia, pharyngitis, rhinititis, sinusitis, URI, rash	Hepatitis, jaundice, GI bleeding, GI perforation, melena, allergic reactions, Liver function test abnormalities, aggravated hypertension, CHF, MI, anemia, acute renal failure, interstitial nephritis, erythema, multiform (rare), Stevens-Johnson syndrome (rare), toxic epidermal necrolysis, exfoliative dermatitis.
Ketorolac **Drugs** **Contraindicated:** Probenicid	Traetment of pain, seasonal allergic conjunctivitis (ophthalmic product), cataract extraction (post-ophthalmic product), incisional referactive surgery (post-ophthalmic product)	Advise not to take aspirin while being treated with this medicine unless advised by doctor or products that contain aspirin, naproxen, or ibuprofen. This medicine may cause drowsiness and may increae the effects of alcohol if affected. Advise the patient that if affected, not to drive a motor vehicle or operate machinery.	Advise to take the tablets with full glass of water	Transient stinging and burning (ophthalmic ketorolac), corneal edema, iritis, ocular irritation, diarrhea, keratitis (ophthalmic ketorolac), edema, abdominal pain, constipation, rash, flatulence, nausea, dizziness, purpura,	Bleeding complications (rare), corneal erosion (rare), corneal perforation (rare), corneal thinning (rare), pallor, epithelial breakdown (rare), palpitations, syncope, liver function test abnormalities, hepatitis, jaundice, GI

Table 1.4 Contd…

Drug	Clinical applications	Cautionary instructions	Dosing in relation to food	Side Effects	
				Common/Mild	Rare/serious
				vomiting, stomatitis, hypertension, injection site pain, pruritis, drowsiness, headache, sweating	bleeding(rare), GI perforation (rare), melena (rare), hearing loss, pancreatitis (rare), hematuria, proteinuria, interstitial nephritis, anemia, leucopenia, thrombocytopenia, angioedema (rare), Steven-johnson syndrome (rare), bronchospasm (rare), aseptic meningitis (rare), convulsions (rare), psychosis (rare).
Mefenamic acid Drugs Contraindicated: N/A	Treatment of analgesic and anti-inflammatory agent	Advise not to take aspirin while being treated with this medicine unless advised by doctor. This medicine may affect mental alertness and or co-rdination. Advise the patient that if affected, not to drive a motor vehicle or operate machinery.	Advise to take with food	Nausea, stomch pain, heartburn, drowsiness or dizziness, blurred vision, weight gain or retaining water.	Rash or hives swelling of face or around eyes, chest tigtness or trouble breathing, sore throat or fever, unusal bleeding or brushing, yellowing of skin or eyes, decreased amount of urine, severe stomach pain or bloody vomit, bloody or black tarry stools, diarrhea.

Table 1.4 Contd...

Drug	Clinical applications	Cautionary instructions	Dosing in relation to food	Side Effects	
				Common/Mild	Rare/serious
Meloxicam **Drugs** **Contraindicated:** N/A	Treatment of osteoarthritis	Caution in case of renal failure unless receiving dialysis, in severe hepatic failure and in bleeding disorders. Adivise not to take aspirin while being treated with this medicine unless advised by doctor.	Advise to take with or after food or milk.	Abdominal pain, diarrhea, rash, URI, UTI, anemia, dyspepsia, flatulence, nausea, edema, dizziness, back pain, headache, insomnia, pharyngitis, arthralgia	Allergic reaction, anaphylaxis, angina, CHF, hypertension, MI, vasculitis, GI ulceration, GI perforation, melena, pancreatitis, arrhythmias, agranulocytosis, leucopenia, purpura, thrombocytopenia, liver function test abnormalities,
Rofecoxib **Drugs** **Contraindicated:** N/A	Treatment of osteoarthritis, migraine headache with or without aura, pain, primary dysmenorrheal, rheumatoid arthritis	Rofecoxib was voluntarily withdrawn from U.S. and world wide market September 30, 2004 due to safety concern of an increased risk for cardiovascular events including heart attack and stroke in patients taking rofecoxib.			
Valdecoxib **Drugs** **Contraindicated:** Avoid if hypersensitivity to aspirin or other NSAIDs	Treatment of osteoarthritis, primary dysmenorrheal, rheumatoid arthritis	Caution in case of stomach ulcer, asthma, kidney disease, heart disease, or liver disease.	Advise to take after food	Abdominal pain, diarrhea, dyspepsia, flatulence, nausea, hypertension, back pain, myalgias, peripheral edema, rash, sinusitis, URI, dizziness, headache.	Aggravated hypertension, angina pectoris, arrhythmias, CHF, thrombosis, MI, unstable angina, GI ulceration, GI perforation, anemia, thrombocytopenia, LFT elevations, hepatitis, acute renal failure, anaphylaxis (rare), Stevens-Johnson syndrome (rare), toxic epi-dermal necrolysis (rare).

Chapter 2

Carboxyclic Acid Derivatives

Aspirin

History

Aspirin is a product of the late-nineteenth-century laboratory, pharmaceutical industry, and medical community. The prevailing scientific techniques, industrial approaches, and medical beliefs were instrumental in the development, promotion and reception of the drug. As a result, the present account does not extend further back than a few decades prior to the release of aspirin from the laboratories of Farbenfabriken vormals Friedrich Bayer & Co. in 1899. In contrast, much of the current literature on aspirin attempts to trace the compound back to antiquity through the Ebers papyrus, the Hippocratic writings, and the works of Galen. Such histories tell a simple, linear tale of the numerous "discoveries" proposed to have led to the use of certain salicylate-containing plants, such as willow bark and wintergreen, or salicylate-related compounds, including salicilin and salicylic acid, as cures for a variety of ailments. Indeed, according to Mann and Plummer: Both [salicilin and salicylic acid] attacked fever and pain, and their partisans advocated the salicylates use as antiseptics, mouthwashes, and water preservatives for ocean voyages; one important chemist further suggested (erroneously) that sodium salicylate, a chemical relative, would successfully treat scarlet fever, diphtheria, measles, syphilis, cholera, rabies and anthrax.

Description

Aspirin, also known as acetylsalicylic acid, is not a prescription drug. It is sold over the counter in many forms, from the familiar white tablets to chewing gum and rectal suppositories. Coated, chewable, buffered, and extended-release forms are available. Many other over-the counter medications contain aspirin.

Aspirin belongs to a group of drugs called salicylates. Other members of this group include sodium salicylate, choline salicylate, and magnesium salicylate. These drugs are more expensive and no more effective than aspirin; however, they are a little easier on the patient's stomach. Aspirin is quickly absorbed into the bloodstream and provides rapid and relatively long-lasting pain relief. Aspirin in high doses also reduces inflammation. In addition to relieving pain and reducing inflammation, aspirin also lowers fever by acting on the hypothalamus, which is the part of the brain that regulates temperature. The brain then signals the blood vessels to dilate (widen), which allows heat to leave the body more quickly.

Aspirin, one of the first drugs to come into common usage, is still mostly the widely used in the world - approximately 35,000 metric tonnes are produced and consumed annually, enough to make over 100 billion standard aspirin tablets every year.

Aspirin, also known as 'acetylsalicylic acid', has a

Chemical formula $C_9H_8O_4$

Chemical structure of aspirin :

$$\text{COOH} \quad \text{OCOCH}_3$$

Category: Analgesic; antipyretic; antirheumatic; antithrombotic.

Description: Colourless crystals or white, crystalline powder; odourless or almost odourless.

Solubility: Freely soluble in ethanol (95%); soluble in chloroform and in ether; slightly soluble in water.

Storage: Store in tightly-closed containers in a cool, dry place.

Pharmacodynamics

Mechanism of action

The therapy of rheumatism began thousands of years ago with the use of decoctions or extracts of herbs or plants such as willow bark or leaves, most of which turned out to contain salicylates. Vane discovered the mechanism by which aspirin exerts its anti-inflammatory, analgesic and antipyretic actions. He proved that aspirin and other non-steroidal anti-inflammatory drugs (NSAIDs) inhibit the activity of the enzyme now called cyclooxygenase (COX) which leads to the formation of prostaglandins (PGs) that cause inflammation, swelling, pain and fever. However, by inhibiting this key enzyme in PG synthesis, the aspirin-like drugs also prevent the production of physiologically important PGs which protect the stomach mucosa from damage by hydrochloric acid, maintain kidney function and aggregate platelets when required. Twenty years later, with the discovery of a second COX gene, it became clear that there are two isoforms of the COX enzyme. The constitutive isoform, COX-1, supports the beneficial homeostatic functions, whereas the inducible isoform, COX-2, becomes up regulated by inflammatory mediators and its products cause many of the symptoms of inflammatory diseases such as rheumatoid and osteoarthritis.

Pharmacokinetics

Absorption and Distribution

Aspirin is hydrolyzed primarily to salicylic acid in the gut wall and during first-pass metabolism through the liver. Salicylic acid is absorbed rapidly from the stomach, but most of the absorption occurs in the proximal small intestine. Following absorption, salicylate is distributed to most body tissues and fluids, including fetal tissues, breast milk, and the CNS. High concentrations are found in the liver and kidneys. Salicylate is variably bound to serum proteins, particularly albumin.

Metabolism and Elimination

The biotransformation of aspirin occurs primarily in the liver by the microsomal enzyme system with a plasma half-life of approximately 15 minutes; aspirin is rapidly hydrolyzed to salicylate. At low doses, salicylate elimination follows first-order kinetics. The plasma half-life of salicylate is approximately 2 to 3 hours.

Approximately 10% of aspirin is excreted as unchanged salicylate in the urine. The major metabolites excreted in the urine are salicyluric acid (75%), salicyl phenolic glucuronide (10%), salicyl acyl glucuronide (5%), and gentisic and gentisuric acid (less than 1%) each. 80 to 100% of a single dose is excreted in the urine within 24 to 72 hours.

Adverse Drug Reactions

Gastrointestinal reactions : Doses of 1,000 mg per day of aspirin caused gastrointestinal symptoms and bleeding that, in some cases, were clinically significant. In the largest postinfarction study (the Aspirin Myocardial Infarction Study (AMIS) with 4,500 people), the percentage of incidences of gastrointestinal symptoms for the aspirin (1,000 mg of a standard, solid-tablet formulation) and placebo-treated subjects, respectively, were stomach pain (14.5%, 4.4%), heartburn (11.9%, 4.8%), nausea and/or vomiting (7.6%, 2.1%), hospitalization for GI disorder (4.9%, 3.5%).

Cardiovascular and Biochemical : The dosage of 1,000 mg per day of aspirin was associated with small increases in systolic blood pressure (BP) (average 1.5 to 2.1 mm) and diastolic BP (0.5 to 0.6 mm), depending upon whether maximal or last available readings were used. Blood urea nitrogen and uric acid levels were also increased but by less than 1.0 mg percent. Subjects with marked hypertension or renal insufficiency had been excluded from the trial so that the clinical importance of these observations for such subjects or for any subjects treated over more prolonged periods is not known. It is recommended that patients placed on long-term aspirin treatment, even at doses of 300 mg per day, be seen at regular intervals to assess changes in these measurements.

In Transient Ischemic Attacks

At dosages of 1,000 mg or higher of aspirin per day, gastrointestinal side effects include stomach pain, heartburn, nausea and/or vomiting, as well as increased rates of gross gastrointestinal bleeding.

Drug Interactions

Aspirin may increase, decrease, or change the effects of many drugs. Aspirin can increase the toxicity of such drugs as methotrexate and valproic acid. Taken with such blood-thinning drugs as warfarin and dicumarol, aspirin can increase the risk of excessive bleeding. Aspirin counteracts the effects of certain other drugs, including angiotensin-converting enzyme (ACE) inhibitors and beta blockers, which lower blood pressure, and medicines used to treat gout (probenecid and sulfinpyrazone). Blood pressure may drop unexpectedly and cause fainting or dizziness if aspirin is taken along with nitroglycerin tablets. Aspirin may also interact with diuretics, diabetes medications, other nonsteroidal anti-inflammatory drugs (NSAIDs), seizure medications, and steroids. Anyone who is taking these drugs should ask his or her physician whether they can safely take aspirin.

Alcohol : Has a synergistic effect with aspirin in causing gastrointestinal bleeding.

Corticosteroids : Concomitant administration with aspirin may increase the risk of gastrointestinal ulceration and may reduce serum salicylate levels.

Pyrazolone Derivatives (phenylbutazone, oxyphenbutazone, and possibly dipyrone) : Concomitant administration with aspirin may increase the risk of gastrointestinal ulceration.

Nonsteroidal Antiinflammatory Agents: Aspirin is contraindicated in patients who are hypersensitive to nonsteroidal anti-inflammatory agents.

Urinary Alkalinizers : Decrease aspirin effectiveness by increasing the rate of salicylate renal excretion.

Phenobarbital : Decreases aspirin effectiveness by enzyme induction.

Phenytoin : Serum phenytoin levels may be increased by aspirin.

Propranolol : May decrease aspirin's anti-inflammatory action by competing for the same receptors.

Antacids : Enteric Coated Aspirin should not be given concurrently with antacids, since an increase in the pH of the stomach may affect the enteric coating of the tablets.

Dosage and Administration

Usual Adult Dose : Adults and Children 12 years and over: One or two tablets/caplets with water, may be repeated every four hours as necessary up to 12 tablets/caplets a day or as directed by a doctor. Do not give to children under 12 unless directed by a doctor.

Ischemic Stroke : 50-325 mg once a day. Continue therapy indefinitely.

Suspected Acute MI : The initial dose of 160-162.5 mg is administered as soon as an MI is suspected. The maintenance dose of 160-162.5 mg a day is continued for 30 days post-infarction. After 30 days, consider further therapy based on dosage and administration for prevention of recurrent MI.

Prevention of Recurrent MI : 75-325 mg once a day. Continue therapy indefinitely.

Unstable Angina Pectoris : 75-325 mg once a day. Continue therapy indefinitely.

Chronic Stable Angina Pectoris : 75-325 mg once a day. Continue therapy indefinitely.

Rheumatoid Arthritis : The initial dose is 3 g a day in divided doses. Increase as needed for anti-inflammatory efficacy with target plasma salicylate levels of 150-300 g/mL. At high doses (i.e., plasma levels of greater than 200 mg/mL), the incidence of toxicity increases.

Spondyloarthropathies : Up to 4 g per day in divided doses.

Osteoarthritis : Up to 3 g per day in divided doses.

Arthritis and Pleurisy of SLE : The initial dose is 3 g a day in divided doses. Increase as needed for anti-inflammatory efficacy with target plasma salicylate levels of 150-300 g/mL. At high doses (i.e., plasma levels of greater than 200 mg/mL) the incidence of toxicity increases.

Adults

Pain relief or fever reduction : The usual dosage is one to two tablets every three to four hours, up to six times per day.

Risk reduction for stroke : One tablet four times a day or two tablets twice a day.

Risk reduction for heart attack : Aspirin may be used as a first-line treatment for a heart attack. The patient should chew a single uncoated aspirin tablet, since chewing makes it easier for the body to absorb the medication rapidly. Aspirin will not stop a heart attack, and proper emergency care is essential; however, an aspirin tablet may reduce the amount of damage done by the heart attack.

Patients should check with a physician for the proper dose and number of times per week they should take aspirin to reduce the risk of a heart attack. The most common dose for this purpose is a single baby aspirin tablet taken daily. Enteric-coated aspirin is often used, since it reduces the risk of stomach irritation.

Children

Parents should consult the child's physician about the proper dosage for their child's condition.

Brand Name

Disprin, Ecosprin, ASA

Official In

I.P. – OFFICIAL
B.P.– OFFICIAL
U.S.P – OFFICIAL.

Diflunisal

History

Diflunisal, an analgesic anti inflammatory agent developed by Merch Sharp & Dohme Research Laboratories, is the result of an attempt to identify a salicylic acid derivative superior to aspirin with improved potency, tolerance and duration of action. Although diflunisal, as a salicylate, has many pharmacological attributes similar to those of aspirin, its two primary structural differences from the presence of the difluorphenyl group probably enhances its potency and duration of action, and from the absence of the O-acetyl group may account for its significantly lower toxicity. Lacking the

O-acetyl function, diflunisal is incapable of enzyme acetylation. It influences the prostaglandin synthesis pathway differently and has a reduced effect on platelet function when compared with aspirin.

Description

Diflunisal is an odorless, white, crystalline compound melting at 211-213°C. It fluoresces on exposure to short wave length (254 nm) and wavelength (366 nm) ultraviolet light.

Pharmacokinetics

Absorption

Diflunisal after oral administration in dose of 50-500 mg was well absorbed. Peak plasma level of 85-100μg/ml was obtained about two hours after administration. The oral bioavailability was essentially 100% based on urinary recovery after 96 hours. Diflunisal administrated orally with food showed a 20 min time delay and a 16% reduction in peak plasma concentration but the AUC remained unchanged. The time required to reach the steady state was dose dependent increasing from 3-4 days with a 25 mg twice daily dose to 7-9 days with a 500 mg twice daily dose.

Distribution

There is limited information on the distribution of diflunisal in man. It has been shown to be highly bound to plasma proteins in normal subjects (>99%). The apparent volume of distribution was low (0.1 liter/kg) and, in lactating women, its concentration in milk was 2.7% of its concentration in plasma.

Metabolism and Elimination

Elimination is concentration-dependent and considerably dependent upon conjugation with glucuronic acid. About 80-90% of an oral dose is excreted in the urine 72-96 hours following administration, primarily as the phonemic and acyl glucuronides the principal metabolite is the phenolic glucuronide conjugate of diflunisal accounting for 64% of the radioactivity in the urine after does of 50-500 mg of radiolabllled diflunisal. The ester glucuronide conjugate accounts for 20% of urinary radioactivity. Total body clearance is small (7.9 ml/min). Less than 5% of a single does is recovered in the faces from either unabsorbed drug or biliary excretion.

Elimination is dose-dependent. The terminal half-life in plasma ranges from 5 hours for a 50mg. oral dose to 15 hours for a one gram dose.

Drug Interactions

The bioavailability of diflunisal is significantly decreased by aluminum hydroxide gel in fasted subjects. Concomitant administration of aspirin with diflunisal decreases plasma concentrations of diflunisal but this effect may not be of clinical importance, because difunisal is highly bound to plasma portein, it has the potential for interacting with other protein-bound agents. Diflunisal also causes a 25-30% increase in hydrochlorothiazide plasma concentration and a decrease in its urinary excretion.

Benorylate

Description

Benorylate is combination of paracetamol and an ester of aspirin. It is used as an anti-inflammatory and antipyretic medication. In the treatment of childhood fever, it has been shown to be inferior to paracetamol and aspirin taken separately. In addition, because it is converted to aspirin, benorylate is not recommended in children due to concerns about Reye.

Synonyms

Benoriate (BAN, rNN), Benorylate: FAW-76, Fenasprate; win-11450, 4-sAcetamidophery, O-acetlsalcylate.

Molecular formula - $C_{17}H_3NO_5$

Molecular weight - 313.3

Pharmacokinetics

Benorylate is slowly absorbed virtually unchanged from the gastrointestinal tract. Following absorption, benorylate is rapidly metabolized to salicylate and paracetamol. It is excreted mainly as metabolites of salicylic acid and paracetamol in the urine.

Adverse Effect, Treatment, and Precautions

Benorylate may cause nausea, indigestion, heartburn, constipation, drowsiness, diarrhea, and skin rashes have also been reported in some patients. Some have experienced dizziness, tints and defines associated with high blood salicylate concentrations.

Benorylate, like aspirin should not generally be given to children under the age of 12 years because of the risk of Reye's syndrome.

When an overdose of benorylate is suspected, it has been suggested that plasma concentrations of both salicylate and paracetamol should be measured since a normal plasma-paracetamol concentration cannot necessarily be assumed from a normal plasma salicylate measurement.

Uses and Administration

Benorylate is a aspirin-paracetamol ester with analgesic, anti inflammatory, and antipyretic properties. It is used in the treatment of mild to moderate pain and fever. It is also used in osteoarthritis, rheumatoid arthritis. Benorylate is given by mouth. Preferably after food, in doses of 2 g twice daily for mild to moderate pain and fever. In active rheumatoid arthritis 4 g twice daily may be required. In elderly patients reduced doses of 2 g twice daily or passively 2 g in the morning and 4 g at night should be given a maximum daily dose of 6 g should be exceeded.

Salsalate

History

The use of salicylates dates back to the 19th century. Salsalate was employed as an antipyretic-antirheumatic agent in 1905. The uricosuric properties of salsalate were noted before 1925, and its use continued through 1950, as late as 1965 it was used for a long term treatment of gout.

Description

Salsalate is a nonsteroidal anti- inflammatory agent for oral administration. Chemically salsalate, (salicylsalicylic acid or 2-hydroxybenzolacid 2carboxyphenyl ester) is a dimer of salicylic acid; its structural formula is shown below.

Structural formula

Molecular formula - $C_{14}H_{10}O_5$

Molecular weight - 258.2

Melting point - 148-149

Synonyms

2-((2-Hydroxybenzoyl) oxy) benzoic acid, 2-Carboxyphenol, 2-Carboxyphenyl salicylate, 2-carboxyphenyl ester, Diacesal, Diplosal, Disalcid, Disalcid (TN), Disalicylic acid, Disalyl, Nobacid, O-Salicylcylsalicylsaeure, PersistinSal, EsterSal.

Pharmacodynamics

Mode of action

Non-steroidal anti-inflammatory drugs exert their major therapeutic and adverse effects by inhibition of prostanoid synthesis. Also the interactions with antihypertensive drugs and lithium are caused by this mechanism of action. Cyclo oxygenation is a key enzymatic step in the synthesis of prostanoids. In 1990, 2 isoforms of the enzyme cyclooxygenase have been identified: Prostanoids synthesized by the constitutive cyclooxygenase (COX-1) are involved in physiological homeostasis. In contrast, the inducible cyclooxygenase (COX-2) produces large amounts of prostanoids, mainly contributing to the pathophysiological process of inflammation.

A drug with selectivity for COX-2 would inhibit proinflammatory prostanoid synthesis while sparing physiologic prostanoid synthesis. Thus, a selective COX-2 inhibitor should be anti-inflammatory with less or no gastrointestinal or other NSAID-typical adverse effects. The experiences with currently used NSAID, which show an increasing incidence of side effects as COX-1 inhibition increases, and studies with the COX-2 selective NSAID salsalate and meloxicam, which have less adverse effects than nonselective COX inhibitors. Newly developed drugs with a very high selectivity for COX-2 have now been tested in clinical trials. So far the results suggest that selective and highly selective COX-2 inhibitors have significantly fewer gastrointestinal and renal adverse effects and do not inhibit platelet aggregation.

Pharmacokinetics

Absorption

Salsalate is insoluble in acid gastric fluids (< 0.1 mg/ml at pH 1.0), but readily soluble in the small intestine where it is partially hydrolyzed to two molecules of salicylic acid. A significant portion of the parent compound is absorbed unchanged and undergoes rapid esterase hydrolysis in the body. Salsalate was promptly absorbed (mean time to peak level 1.5 hours)

Distribution

Salsalate did not accumulate in the plasma during multiple dosing. Plasma levels of salicylic acid following single and multiple doses indicate that salsalate is extensively hydrolyzed to salicylic acid in the body. The slightly lower levels of salicylic acid after salsalate than after aspirin may reflect direct biotransformation of some of the salsalate to an salsalate conjugate, without hydrolysis to salicylic acid.

Metabolism

It is a salicylate derivative; on hydrolysis it yields two molecules of salicylic acid, approximately 7-10% of the dose is not hydrolyzed to salicylic acid and appears in the urine either as unchanged drug or glucuronide conjugates. Thus, it is eliminated from plasma with a mean half-life of 1.1 hour. Less than 1 per cent was excreted in the urine as unchanged salsalate.

Elimination

About 13% is excreted through the kidney as a glucuronide conjugate of the parent compound, the remainder as salicylic acid and its metabolites. Thus, the amount of salicylic acid available from salsalate is about 15% less than from aspirin, when the two drugs are administered on a salicylic acid molar equivalent basis (3.6gm salsalate/5gm aspirin). Salsalate was excreted primarily in the urine only approximately 1% of the total dose was found in the stools the incomplete availability of salicylate from salsalate that has been previously reported may not be due to incomplete absorption of the drug but to incomplete hydrolysis to salicylic acid.

Drug Interactions

Salicylates antagonize the uricosuric action of Drugs used to treat gout. Aspirin and other salicylate drug will be additive to disalcid and may increase plasma concentrations of salicylic acid to toxic levels. Drugs and foods that raise urine pH will increase renal clearance and urinary excretion of salicylic acid, thus lowering plasma levels; acidifying drugs or foods will decrease urinary excretion and increase plasma levels. Salicylates given concomitantly with anticoagulant drugs may predispose to systemic bleeding. Salicylates may enhance the hypoglycemic effect of oral anti diabetic drugs of the sulfonylurea class. Salicylate competes with a number of drugs for protein binding sites, notably penicillin, thiopental. If Disalcid is taken with certain other drugs, the effects of either could be increased, decreased, or altered. It is especially important to check before combining salsalate with the following:-

Alcohol, Antacids (in large doses), Anti-inflammatory drugs (NSAIDs, such as ibuprofen), Hormones such as prednisone or cortisone, Medicines used to treat or prevent blood clots, Medicines for diabetes that are taken orally, Medicines for gout, Methotrexate, Seizure (convulsion) or epilepsy medicine, Acetazolamide (Diamox), Bufferin and Empirin and Blood-thinning medications such as Coumadin.

Adverse Drug Reactions

- Allergic reaction: Itching or hives, swelling in face or hands, Swelling or tingling in mouth or throat, chest tightness, trouble breathing.
- Bloody or black, tarry stools.
- Change in how much or how often urinate.
- Chest pain, shortness of breath, or coughing up blood.
- Dark-colored urine or pale stools.
- Flu-like symptoms.
- Pain in lower leg (calf).
- Problems with vision, speech, or walking.
- Rapid weight gain.
- Ringing in ears.
- Severe stomach pain.
- Shortness of breath, cold sweat, and bluish-colored skin.
- Skin rash or blisters with fever.
- Sudden or severe headache.
- Vomiting blood or something that looks like coffee grounds.

Drug abuse and dependence

Drug abuse and dependence have not been reported with salsalate.

Drug/ Laboratory Test Interactions

Salicylate competes with thyroid hormone for binding to plasma proteins, which may be reflected in a depressed plasma T_4 value in some patients; thyroid function and basal metabolism are unaffected.

Dosage and Administration

Two doses of three 500 mg tablets/capsules; or Three doses of two 500 mg tablets/capsules.

Some patients, e.g., the elderly, may require a lower dosage to achieve therapeutic blood concentrations and to avoid the more common side effects such as auditory. Alleviation of symptoms is gradual, and full benefit may not be evident for 3 to 4 days, when plasma salicylate levels have achieved steady state. There is no evidence for development of tissue tolerance (tachyphylaxis).

Adults

The usual dosage is 3,000 milligrams daily, divided into smaller doses as follows:

1. 2 doses of two 750-milligram tablets, or
2. 2 doses of three 500-milligram tablets or capsules, or
3. 3 doses of two 500-milligram tablets or capsules

Children

Dosage recommendations and indications for use in children have not been established.

Older adults

A lower dosage may be sufficient to achieve desired blood levels without the more common side effects.

Contraindications

- Anemia
- Bleeding or clotting problems
- Drink more than 3 alcohol-containing beverages a day
- Gout
- Heart disease, including heart failure
- High blood pressure
- Kidney disease
- Liver disease
- Smoking tobacco
- Stomach ulcers, or other stomach problems
- Systemic lupus erythematosus (SLE)

- Thrombotic thrombocytopenic purpuria (TTP)
- Ulcerative colitis
- Vitamin K deficiency
- Pregnant or trying to get pregnant
- Breast-feeding

Warnings

Reye's syndrome may develop in individuals who have chicken pox, influenza, or flu symptoms. Some studies suggest a possible association between the development of Reye's syndrome and the use of medicines containing salicylate or aspirin. Salsalate contains a salicylate and therefore is not recommended for use in patients with chicken pox, influenza, or flu symptoms.

Precautions

General

Patients on treatment with salsalate should be warned not to take other salicylates so as to avoid potentially toxic concentrations. Great care should be exercised when it is prescribed in the presence of chronic renal insufficiency or peptic ulcer disease. Protein binding of salicylic acid can be influenced by nutritional status, competitive binding of other drugs, and fluctuations in serum proteins caused by disease (rheumatoid arthritis, etc.). Although cross reactivity, induding bronchospasm, has been reported occasionally with non-acetylated salicylates, including salsalate, in aspirin-sensitive patients, salsalate is less likely than aspirin to induce asthma in such patients.

Laboratory Tests

Plasma salicylic acid concentrations should be periodically monitored during long term treatment with salsalate to aid maintenance of therapeutically effective levels: 10 to 30 mg/100 ml. Toxic manifestations are not usually seen until plasma concentrations exceed 30 mg/l00 ml. Urinary pH should also be regularly monitored: sudden acidification, as from pH 6.5 to 5.5, cans double the plasma level, resulting in toxicity.

Use in Pregnancy

Pregnancy Category C

Salsalate and salicylic acid have been shown to be teratogenic and embryocidal in rats when given in doses 4 to 5 times the usual human dose.

The effects were not observed at doses twice as great as the usual human dose. There are no adequate and well-controlled studies in pregnant women. Salsalate should be used during pregnancy only if the potential benefit justifies the potential risk to the fetus.

Pediatric Use

Safety and effectiveness in pediatric patients have not been established.

Therapeutic uses

Salsalate is indicated for relief of the signs and symptoms of rheumatoid arthritis, osteoarthritis and related rheumatic disorders. Salsalate is also used to relieve mild pain, to reduce fever, and to reduce the pain and inflammation (swelling) caused by arthritis or other inflammatory conditions.

Brand names

Argesic, Disalcid, Mono-gesic, Salfex, Salsitab, Marthritic, Amigesic, Anaflex 750

Sodium Salicylate

History

The use of salicylates dates back to the 19th century. Sodium salicylate was employed as an antipyretic-antirheumatic agent in 1875. The uricosuric properties of sodium salicylate were noted before 1890, and its use continued through 1950, as late as 1955 it was used for long term treatment of gout.

Description

Synonyms

Sodium 2-hydroxy benzoate, saliglutin, Enterosalil, 2-hydroxy- monosodium salt, Enterosalicyl, Enterosalil, Entrosalyl, Glutosalyl, Natrium salicylat, Neo-salicyl, o-Hydroxybenzoic acid monosodium salt.

Standards

Sodium salicylate contains not less than 99.0 per cent and not more than 101.0 per cent of $C_7H_5NaO_3$, calculated with reference to the dried substance.

> **Molecular formula -** $C_7H_5NaO_3$
>
> **Molecular weight -** 160.10

Structural formula

$$\text{COONa} \quad \text{OH}$$

Category : Anti-inflammatory; analgesic.

Dose : 500 mg to 2 g, with food; in the treatment of acute rheumatism, 5 to 10 g daily, in divided doses.

Solubility : Freely soluble in water (concentrated solutions are liable to deposit crystals of the hexahydrate) and in ethanol (95%); practically insoluble in ether.

Storage : Store in tightly-closed, light-resistant containers.

Pharmacodynamics

Mechanism of action

Sodium salicylate inhibited prostaglandin E_2 release when added together with interleukin-1 for 24 hr with an IC_{50} value of 5 μg/ml, an effect that was independent of NF-B activation or COX-2 transcription or translation. Sodium salicylate acutely (30 min) also caused a concentration-dependent inhibition of COX-2 activity measured in the presence of 0, 1, or 10 μM exogenous arachidonic acid. In contrast, when exogenous arachidonic acid was increased to 30 μM, sodium salicylate was a very weak inhibitor of COX-2 activity with an IC_{50} of >100 μg/ml. Thus, sodium salicylate is an effective inhibitor of COX-2 activity at concentrations far below those required to inhibit NF-B (20 mg/ml) activation and is easily displaced by arachidonic acid.

Action of sodium salicylate on tissue metabolism in vitro

Sodium salicylate, uncouple oxidative phosphorylation in liver, kidney and brain mitochondrial preparations. Liver and kidney are more sensitive to this agent than is brain. The uncoupling action is qualitatively similar to that seen with the classical uncoupling agent, 2, 4-dinitro-phenol. The concentrations of salicylates used in these studies are comparable to toxic levels in the intact animal.

These compounds stimulate the oxygen consumption of brain mitochondria in an ortho phosphate and acceptor-saturated system, with pyruvate and malate as substrate. This effect is not abolished by incubation of brain mitochondria with ethylenediaminetetraacetate. Sodium salicylates stimulate the respiratory rate of an acceptor-deficient system and inhibit fatty acid oxidation of rat liver mitochondria. Like dinitrophenol, these agents enhance the liberation of inorganic phosphate from ATP.

Sodium salicylate, effectively depress oxidative phosphorylation and the oxygen consumption of liver and muscle slices from salicylate treated-rats is increased. It is suggested that the above actions are responsible for many of the manifestations of salicylate poisoning.

Adverse Drug Reaction

When sodium salicylate is used in the treatment of rheumatic fever its high sodium content may cause problems in patient with cardiac complications. The use of this drug is generally not recommended for children under the age of 12 years because of the risk of Reye's syndrome, unless specifically indicated.

Dosages and Administration

- For oral dosage forms (tablets or delayed-release [enteric-coated] tablets):

  For pain or fever

- Adults and teenagers-325 or 650 milligrams (mg) every four hours as needed.

- Children up to 6 years of age-This medicine is too strong for use in children younger than 6 years of age.

- Children 6 years of age and older-325 mg every four hours as needed.

  For arthritis

- Adults and teenagers-A total of 3600 to 5400 mg a day, divided into several smaller doses.

- Children-A total of 80 to 100 mg per kilogram (kg) (32 to 40 mg per pound) of body weight a day, divided into several smaller doses.

Therapeutic Uses

Sodium salicylate is used as analgesic anti–inflammatory and for antipyretic actions. It is also used in the treatment of pain, fever, and in rheumatic arthritis. It is also used in the symptomatic treatment of rheumatic fever. It is applied topically in concentrations usually ranging from 1 to about 6% as a keratolytic. Up to 60% is used as a caustic in preparations for removal of warts.

Trisalicylate

(Choline magnesium trisalicylate)

Description

Trisalicylate are nonsteroidal, anti-inflammatory preparations containing choline magnesium trisalicylate which is freely soluble in water. The absolute structure of choline magnesium trisalicylate is not known at this time.

Molecular formula - $C_{26}H_{29}O_{10}NMg$

Chemical formula & Structure - $C_{21}H_{12}O_6$

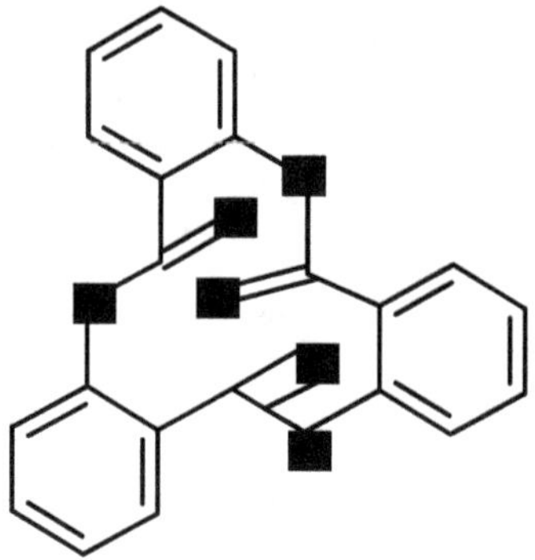

Molecular weight - 539.8

Solubility : This substance when dissolved in water would appear to form 5 ions (1 choline ion, 1 magnesium ion and 3 salicylate ions).

Pharmacokinetics

Trisalicylate Tablets/Liquid contain salicylate with anti-inflammatory, analgesic and antipyretic action. On ingestion of Trisalicylate tablets/ liquid, the salicylate moiety is absorbed rapidly and reaches peak blood levels within an average of one to two hours after single doses of the tablets or liquid.

The primary route of excretion is renal; the excretion products are chiefly the glycine and glucuronide conjugates. At higher serum salicylate concentrations, the glycine conjugation pathway becomes rapidly saturated. Thus, the slower glucuronide conjugation pathway becomes the rate limiting step for salicylate excretion. In addition, salicylate excreted in the bile as glucuronide conjugate may be reabsorbed. These factors account for the prolongation of salicylate half-life and the nonlinear increase in plasma salicylate level as the salicylate dose is increased. The serum concentration of salicylate is increased by conditions that decrease glomerular filtration rate or proximal tubular secretion.

The bioequivalence of Trisalicylate Liquid and Tablets 500 mg/ 750 mg/ 1000 mg has been established. With the tablets, a steady-state condition is usually reached after 4 to 5 doses, and the half- life of elimination, on repeated administration of tablets, is 9 to 17 hours. This permits a maintenance dosage schedule of once or twice daily. Unlike aspirin and certain other non-steroidal anti-inflammatory agents, such as aryl propionic acid derivatives and aryl acetic acid derivatives, choline magnesium trisalicylate, at therapeutic dosage levels, does not affect platelet aggregation, as shown by *in vitro* and *in vivo* studies.

Drug Interactions

- Foods and drugs that alter urine pH may affect renal clearance of salicylate and plasma salicylate concentrations.

- Raising urine pH, as with chronic antacid use, can enhance renal salicylate clearance and diminish plasma salicylate concentration; urine acidification can decrease urinary salicylate excretion and increase plasma levels.

- When salicylate drug products are concurrently dosed with other plasma protein bound drug products, adverse effects may result.

- Caution should be exercised in administering trisalicylate to rheumatoid arthritis patients on methotrexate.

- The efficacy of uricosuric agents may be decreased when administered with salicylate products.

- Larger salicylate doses (over 5 grams per day) can induce uricosuria and lower plasma urate levels.

- Corticosteroids can reduce plasma salicylate levels by increasing renal elimination and perhaps by also stimulating hepatic metabolism of salicylates.

Adverse Drug Reactions

Gastrointestinal: nausea, heartburn, stomach pains, dyspepsia, epigastria, discomfort.

Indications

Osteoarthritis, Rheumatoid Arthritis and Acute Painful Shoulder.

Salicylates are considered the base therapy of choice in the arthrities; and trisalicylate preparations are indicated for the relief of the signs and symptoms of rheumatoid arthritis, osteoarthritis and other arthrities. Trisalicylate tablets or liquid is indicated in the long-term management of these diseases and especially in the acute flare of rheumatoid arthritis. Trisalicylate tablets or liquid is also indicated for the treatment of acute painful shoulder.

Trisalicylate preparations are effective and generally well tolerated, and are logical choices whenever salicylate treatment is indicated. They are particularly suitable when a once-a-day or b.i.d. dosage regimen is important to patient compliance; when gastrointestinal intolerance to aspirin is encountered; when gastrointestinal micro bleeding or hematological effects of aspirin are considered a patient hazard; and when interference (or the risk of interference) with normal platelet function by aspirin or by propionic acid derivatives is considered to be clinically undesirable. Use of trisalicylate liquid is appropriate when a liquid dosage form is preferred, as in the elderly patient.

Dosage and Administration

Adults

In rheumatoid arthritis, osteoarthritis, the more severe arthritis, and acute painful shoulder, the recommended starting dosage is 1500 mg given b.i.d. Some patients may be treated with 3000 mg given once per day (h.s.) In the elderly patient, a daily dosage of 2250 mg given as 750 mg t.i.d. may be efficacious and well tolerated. Dosage should be adjusted in accordance with the patient's response. In patients with renal dysfunction, monitor salicylate levels and adjust dose accordingly.

For mild to moderate pain or for antipyresis, the usual dosage is 2000 mg to 3000 mg daily in divided doses (b.i.d.). Based on patient response or salicylate blood levels, dosage may be adjusted to achieve optimum therapeutic effect. Salicylate blood levels should be in the range of 15 to 30 mg/ 100 mL for anti-inflammatory effect and 5 to 15 mg/ 100 mL for analgesia and antipyresis.

Children

Usual daily dose for children for anti- inflammatory or analgesic action:

Trisalicylate 500 mg Tablets/Liquid and Trisalicylate 750 mg and 1000mg Tablets, 50 mg/kg/day.

Overdose

Death in adults has been reported following ingestion of doses from 10 to 30 grams of salicylate; however, larger doses have been taken without resulting fatality. Symptoms of overdose include tinnitus, vomiting, acute renal failure, hyperthermia, irritability, seizures, coma, and metabolic acidosis. For acute ingestion, determine serum salicylate levels 6 hours after ingestion.

Symptoms

Salicylate intoxication, known as salicylism, may occur with large doses or extended therapy. Common symptoms of salicylism include headache, dizziness, tinnitus, hearing impairment, confusion, drowsiness, sweating, vomiting, diarrhea, and hyperventilation. A more severe degree of salicylate intoxication can lead to CNS disturbances, alteration in electrolyte balance, respiratory and metabolic acidosis, hyperthermia, and dehydration.

Treatment

Reduction of further absorption of salicylate from the gastrointestinal tract can be achieved via emesis, gastric lavage, use of activated charcoal, or a combination of the above. Appropriate I.V. fluids should be administered to correct dehydration, electrolyte imbalance, and acidosis and to maintain adequate renal function. To accelerate salicylate excretion, forced diuresis with alkalinizing solution is recommended. In extreme cases, peritoneal dialysis or hemodialysis should be considered for effective salicylate removal.

Side Effects

Tinnitus, gastrointestinal complaints, nausea, vomiting, gastric upset, indigestion, heartburn, diarrhea, epigastric pain, headache, lightheadedness, dizziness, drowsiness, lethargy.

Use in Pregnancy

Pregnancy Category C

Animal reproduction studies have not been conducted with trisalicylate preparations. It is also not known whether trisalicylate can cause fetal harm when administered to a pregnant woman or can affect reproduction capacity. Trisalicylate should be given to a pregnant woman only if clearly needed. Because of the known effects of other salicylate drug products on the fetal cardiovascular system (closure of ductus arteriosus), use during late pregnancy should be avoided.

Labor and Delivery

The effects of trisalicylate on labor and delivery in pregnant women are unknown. Since prolonged gestation and prolonged labor due to prostaglandin inhibition have been reported with the use of other salicylate products, the use of trisalicylate preparations near term is not recommended. Other salicylate products have also been associated with alterations in maternal and neonatal hemostasis mechanisms and with perinatal mortality.

Nursing Mothers

Salicylate is excreted in human milk. Peak milk salicylate levels are delayed, occurring as long as 9 to 12 hours post dose, and the milk: plasma ratio has been reported to be as high as 0.34. Because of the potential for significant salicylate absorption by the nursing infant, caution should be exercised when trisalicylate is administered to a nursing woman.

Therapeutic Uses

- Management of osteoarthritis.
- Rheumatoid arthritis and other arthritis.
- Analgesic and Antipyretic Action.
- Anti- inflammatory or analgesic action.
- Juvenile rheumatoid arthritis and other appropriate conditions.

Brand Names

    In India: - cmt, tricosal, trilisate

    In U.S.A.:- trilisate

Aceclofenac

Description

Aceclofenac is an orally administered phenyl acetic acid derivatives with effects on a variety of inflammatory mediators. Aceclofenac contains not less than 99.0% and not more than the equivalent of 101.0 percent of 2-[[2-[2-[(2, 6-dichlorophenyl) amino] phenyl] acetyl] oxy] acetic acid.

It is a white or almost white crystalline powder. It is an effective analgesic and anti-inflammatory agent with a good tolerability profile. Through its analgesic and anti-inflammatory properties, aceclofenac provides symptomatic relief in a variety of painful conditions. A reduction in the stimulated generation of reactive oxygen species (O_2), which may play a role in joint damage, was observed after 15 days in these patients, but after

180 days. At day 180, O_2 release was similar to that seen in a group of 41 healthy untreated individuals.

Aceclofenac has been shown to have potent analgesic and anti-inflammatory activities, similar to indomethacin and diclofenac and due to its preferential COX-2 blockade it has better safety than conventional NSAIDs with respect to adverse effects on gastrointestinal and cardiovascular system.

IUPAC Name - {[2-(2',6'-dichlorophenyl)amino]phenylacetoxyacetic acid}

Formula - $C_{16}H_{13}NCl_2O_4$

Mol Weight - 354.2 g/mol

Chemistry

Aceclofenac (ACF), {[2-(2', 6'-dichlorophenyl) amino] phenyl acetoxyacetic acid} is a new phenyl acetic acid derivative with potent analgesic and antiinflammatory properties and improved gastric tolerance. Paracetamol (PCM), chemically 4-hydroxy acetanilide, is a centrally and peripherally acting analgesic and antipyretic agent. Several combination dosage forms of these two drugs containing ACF (100 mg) and PCM (500 mg) are available commercially. This combination is used for pain relief and management of rheumatoid arthritis.

Aceclofenac, a phenylacetic acid derivative is peripherally acting, non-steroidal anti-inflammatory analgesic with anti-inflammatory, antiarthritic and antipyretic activities. It is converted to active metabolites intracellularly that inhibit the production of prostaglandins. Aceclofenac demonstrates better gastric tolerance and consequently offers greater potential security than other NSAIDs such as indomethacin and diclofenac.

Structure Activity Relationship

Structure-activity relationship in this series, have not been extensively studied. It does appear that the function of the two o-chloro groups is to force the anilino-phenyl ring out of the plane of the phenylacetic acid portion, this twisting effect being important in the binding of NSAIDs to the active site of the cyclooxygenase enzyme

Pharmacodynamics

Mechanism of action

Aceclofenac belongs to a group of medicines called non-steroidal anti-inflammatory drugs (NSAIDs). It works by blocking the action of a substance in the body called cyclo-oxygenase. Cyclo-oxygenase is involved in the production of various chemicals in the body, some of which are known as prostaglandins. Prostaglandins are produced in response to injury or certain diseases and would otherwise go on to cause pain, swelling and inflammation. Arthritic conditions are one example of this. Aceclofenac is used to relieve pain and inflammation in arthritic conditions. All the medicines in this group reduce inflammation caused by the body's own immune system and are effective pain killers.

Pharmacokinetics

Aceclofenac is rapidly and completely absorbed after oral administration, peak plasma concentrations are reached 1 to 3 hours after an oral dose. The drug is highly protein bound (7.99%). The presence of food does alter the extent of absorption of aceclofenac but the absorption rate is reduced. The plasma concentration of aceclofenac was approximately twice that in synovial fluid after multiple doses of the drug in-patient with knee pain and synovial fluid effusion. Aceclofenac is metabolized to a major metabolite, 4'-hydroxyaceclofenac and to a number of other metabolites including 5 hydroxyaceclofenac, 4'-hydroxydiclofenac, diclofenac and 5-hydroxy-diclofenac. Renal excretion is the main route of elimination of aceclofenac with 70 to 80% of an administered dose found in the urine, mainly as the glucuronides of aceclofenac and its metabolites of each dose of aceclofenac, 20% is excreted in the faeces. The plasma elimination half-life of the drug is approximately 4 hours.

Drug Interactions

Aceclofenac may increase plasma concentrations of lithium, digoxin and methotrexate, increase the activity of anticoagulant, inhibit the activity of diuretics, enhance cyclosporin nephrotoxicity and precipitate convulsions when co-administered with quinolone antibiotics. Furthermore, hypo or hyperglycaemia may result from the concomitant administration of aceclofenac and antidiabetic drugs, although this is rare. The co administration of aceclofenac with other NSAIDS or corticosteroids may results in increased frequency of adverse event.

Side Effect

Headache, rash, excess gas in the stomach and intestines (flatulence), disturbed sleep, blood disorders, disturbances of the gut such as diarrhoea, constipation, nausea, vomiting or abdominal pain indigestion (dyspepsia) balance problems involving the inner ear (vertigo), dizziness, excessive fluid retention in the body tissues, resulting in swelling (oedema) difficulty in breathing (dyspnoea), inflammation of the lining of the mouth (stomatitis), itching (pruritis), inflammation of the skin (dermatitis), inflammation of the stomach (gastritis), alteration in results of liver function tests.

Adverse Drug Reaction

Aceclofenac is well tolerated, with most adverse events being minor and reversible and affecting mainly the GI system. Most common events include dyspepsia (7.5%), abdominal pain (6.2%), nausea (1.5%), diarrhea (1.5%), flatulence (0.8%), gastritis (0.6%), constipation (0.5%), vomiting (0.5%), ulcerative stomatitis (0.1%), pancreatitis (0.1%).

Although the incidence of gastro intestinal adverse events with aceclofenac was similar to those of comparator NSAIDS in individual clinical trials, withdrawal rates due to these events were significantly lower aceclofenac than with ketoprofen and tenoxicam. Other adverse effect, which is not common such as dizziness (1%), vertigo (0.3%), and rare cases: paraesthesia and tremor.

Dosage and Administration

The usual dose of aceclofenac is 100 mg given twice daily by mouth, one tablet in the morning and one in the evening. There is no evidence that the dosage of aceclofenac needs to be modified in patients with mild renal impairment, but as with other NSAIDs caution should be exercised.

Clinical Efficacy

In large trials of 2 to 6 months duration, aceclofenac significantly reduced pain and improves functional capacity and mobility relative to baseline in patients with osteoarthritis, rheumatoid arthritis or ankylosing spondylitis and reduces inflammation in patients with rheumatoid arthritis. No head to head comparison between aceclofenac and coxibs have been performed, nor for efficacy neither for tolerance.

Therapeutic Uses

In osteoarthritis, in rheumatoid arthritis, in ankylosing spondylitis, in dental pain, in postoperative pain, in Dysmenorrhoea, in acute lumbago, in musculoskeletal trauma, Gonalgia (Knee pain)

Brand Names

India_– Hi Fenac, fena plus

Diclofenac

Description

Diclofenac is a NSAIDs taken to reduce inflammation and an analgesic reducing pain in conditions such as in arthritis or acute injury. It can also be used to reduce menstrual pain.

Diclofenac is well-tolerated after 30 years experience by the general human population, but may unexpectedly become intolerated in some of the elderly population of long term users.

Structural formula

IUPAC Name - 2-[2-(2,6-dichlorophenyl) aminophenyl]ethanoic acid

Formula - $C_{14}H_{11}NCl_2O_2$

Mol Weight - 296.148 g/mol

Pharmacodynamics

Mechanism of action

The action of one single dose is much longer (6 to 8 hours) than the very short half-life of the drug indicates. This could partly be due to a particular high concentration achieved in synovial fluids. The exact mechanism of action is not entirely known, but it is thought that the primary mechanism responsible for its anti-inflammatory/antipyretic/analgesic action is inhibition of prostaglandin synthesis by inhibition of cyclooxygenase (COX).

Inhibition of COX also decreases prostaglandins in the epithelium of the stomach, making it more sensitive to corrosion by gastric acid. This is also the main side effect of diclofenac. Diclofenac has a low to moderate preference to block the COX2-isoenzyme (approximately 10-fold) and is said to have therefore a somewhat lower incidence of gastrointestinal complaints than noted with indomethacin and aspirin.

Diclofenac may also be a unique member of the NSAIDs. There is some evidence that diclofenac inhibits the lipooxygenase pathways, thus reducing formation of the leukotrienes (also pro-inflammatory autacoids). There is also speculation that diclofenac may inhibit phospholipase A_2 as part of its mechanism of action. These additional actions may explain the high potency of diclofenac-it is the most potent NSAIDs on a molar basis.

There are marked differences among NSAIDs in their selective inhibition of the two subtypes of cyclo-oxygenase, COX-1 and COX-2. Much pharmaceutical drug design has attempted to focus on selective COX-2 inhibition as a way to minimize the gastrointestinal side effects of non-selective NSAIDs like aspirin. In practice, use of some COX-2 inhibitors has led to massive numbers of patient family lawsuits alleging wrongful death by heart attack, yet other significantly COX-selective NSAIDs like diclofenac have been well-tolerated by most of the population.

Pharmacokinetics

Absorption

Diclofenac is 100% absorbed after oral administration compared to IV administration as measured by urine recovery. However, due to first-pass metabolism, only about 50% of the absorbed dose is systemically available. Food has no significant effect on the extent of diclofenac absorption. However, there is usually a delay in the onset of absorption of 1 to 4.5 hours and a reduction in peak plasma levels of <20%.

Distribution

The apparent volume of distribution (V/F) of diclofenac sodium is 1.4 L/kg. Diclofenac is more than 99% bound to human serum proteins, primarily to albumin. Serum protein binding is constant over the concentration range (0.15-105 mcg/mL) achieved with recommended doses. Diclofenac diffuses into and out of the synovial fluid. Diffusion into the joint occurs when plasma levels are higher than those in the synovial fluid, after which the process reverses and synovial fluid levels are higher than plasma levels. It is not known whether diffusion into the joint plays a role in the effectiveness of diclofenac.

Metabolism

Five diclofenac metabolites have been identified in human plasma and urine. The metabolites include 4'-hydroxy-, 5-hydroxy-, 3'-hydroxy-, 4',5-dihydroxy- and 3'-hydroxy-4'-methoxy diclofenac. In patients with renal dysfunction, peak concentrations of metabolites 4'-hydroxy- and 5-hydroxy-diclofenac were approximately 50% and 4% of the parent compound after single oral dosing compared to 27% and 1% in normal healthy subjects. However, diclofenac metabolites undergo further glucuronidation and sulfation followed by biliary excretion. One diclofenac metabolite 4'-hydroxy- diclofenac has very weak pharmacologic activity.

Excretion

Diclofenac is eliminated through metabolism and subsequent urinary and biliary excretion of the glucuronide and the sulfate conjugates of the metabolites. Little or no free unchanged diclofenac is excreted in the urine. Approximately 65% of the dose is excreted in the urine and approximately 35% in the bile as conjugates of unchanged diclofenac plus metabolites. Because renal elimination is not a significant pathway of elimination for unchanged diclofenac, dosing adjustment in patients with mild to moderate renal dysfunction is not necessary. The terminal half-life of unchanged diclofenac is approximately 2 hours.

Bioavailability - 100%

Protein binding - more than 99%

Metabolism - hepatic, no active metabolites exist

Half life - 1.2-2 hr (35% of the drug enters enterohepatic recirculation)

Excretion - biliary, only 1% in urine

Drug Interactions

Aspirin : When diclofenac is administered with aspirin, its protein binding is reduced. The clinical significance of this interaction is not known; however, as with other NSAIDs, concomitant administration of diclofenac and aspirin is not generally recommended because of the potential of increased adverse effects.

Methotrexate : NSAIDs have been reported to competitively inhibit methotrexate accumulation in rabbit kidney slices. This may indicate that they could enhance the toxicity of methotrexate. Caution should be used when NSAIDs are administered concomitantly with methotrexate.

Cyclosporine : Diclofenac, like other NSAIDs, may affect renal prostaglandins and increase the toxicity of certain drugs. Therefore, concomitant therapy with diclofenac may increase cyclosporine nephrotoxicity. Caution should be used when diclofenac is administered concomitantly with cyclosporine.

ACE-inhibitors : NSAIDs may diminish the antihypertensive effect of ACE inhibitors. This interaction should be given consideration in patients taking NSAIDs concomitantly with ACE inhibitors.

Diuretics : Clinical studies, as well as post-marketing observations, have shown that diclofenac can reduce the natriuretic effect of furosemide and thiazides in some patients. This response has been attributed to inhibition of renal prostaglandin synthesis. During concomitant therapy with NSAIDs, the patient should be observed closely for signs of renal failure.

Lithium : NSAIDs have produced an elevation of plasma lithium levels and a reduction in renal lithium clearance. The mean minimum lithium concentration increased 15% and the renal clearance was decreased by approximately 20%. These effects have been attributed to inhibition of renal prostaglandin synthesis by the NSAIDs. Thus, when NSAIDs and lithium are administered concurrently, subjects should be observed carefully for signs of lithium toxicity.

Warfarin : The effects of warfarin and NSAIDs on GI bleeding are synergistic, such that users of both drugs together have a risk of serious GI bleeding higher than users of either drug alone.

Adverse Drug Reaction

Diclofenac is among the better tolerated NSAIDs. 20% of patients on long-term treatment experience side effects, only 2% have to discontinue the drug, mostly due to gastrointestinal complaints. Gastrointestinal complaints are most often noted the development of ulceration and/or bleeding requires immediate termination of treatment with diclofenac. Most patients receive an ulcer-protective drug as prophylaxis during long-term treatment (misoprostol, ranitidine 150mg at bedtime or omeprazole 20 mg at bedtime).

Bone marrow depression is noted infrequently (leukopenia, agranulocytosis, thrombopenia with/without purpura, aplastic anemia). These conditions may be life-threatening and/or irreversible, if detected too late. All patients should be monitored closely. Diclofenac is a weak and reversible inhibitor of thrombocytic aggregation needed for normal coagulation.

Liver and renal damage occur infrequently, but are usually reversible. Hepatitis may occur rarely without any warning symptoms and may be fatal. Patients with osteoarthritis develop more often symptomatic liver disease than patients with rheumatoid arthritis. Liver and kidney function should be monitored regularly during long-term treatment. If used for the short term treatment of pain or fever, diclofenac has not been found to be more hepatotoxic than other NSAIDs.

Contraindications

- Hypersensitivity against diclofenac
- History of allergic reactions (bronchospasm, shock, rhinitis, urticaria) following the use of Aspirin or another NSAIDs
- Third-trimester pregnancy
- Active stomach and/or duodenal ulceration or gastrointestinal bleeding

- Inflammative intestinal disorders such as Crohn's disease or ulcerative colitis
- Severe insufficiency of the heart
- Recently, a warning has been issued by FDA not to treat patients recovering from heart surgery
- Severe liver insufficiency (Child-Pugh Class C)
- Severe renal insufficiency (creatinine clearance <30 ml/min)
- Caution in patients with preexisting hepatic porphyria, as diclofenac may trigger attacks
- Caution in patients with severe, active bleeding such as cerebral hemorrhage

Dosage and Administration

Carefully consider the potential benefits and risks of diclofenac and other treatment options before deciding to use diclofenac. Use the lowest effective dose for the shortest duration consistent with individual patient treatment goals. After observing the response to initial therapy with diclofenac the dose and frequency should be adjusted to suit an individual patient's needs. For the relief of osteoarthritis, the recommended dosage is 100-150 mg/day in divided doses (50 mg b.i.d. or t.i.d., or 75 mg b.i.d.). For the relief of rheumatoid arthritis, the recommended dosage is 150-200 mg/day in divided doses (50 mg t.i.d. or q.i.d., or 75 mg b.i.d.). For the relief of ankylosing spondylitis, the recommended dosage is 100-125 mg/day, administered as 25 mg q.i.d., with an extra 25-mg dose at bedtime if necessary.

Brand Names

India - Voltaren, Voltarol, Diclon Dicloflex Difen, Difene, Cataflam, Rhumalgan and Abitren

U.S.A - Dicloflex and Cataflam

Tolmetin

Description

Sodium 1-methyl-5-(4-methylbenzoyl)-1H-pyrrole-2-acetate dihydrate

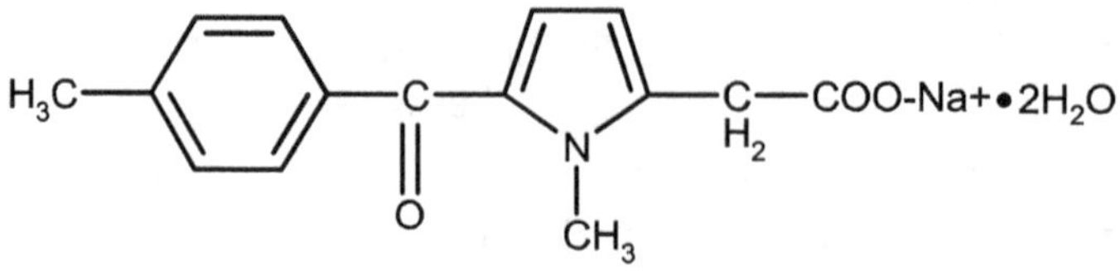

Chemical Formula : $C_{15}H_{14}NNaO_3$, 2H2O

Molecular Weight : 315.3

Pharmacodynamics

The mode of action for tolmetin is not known. However, studies in laboratory animals and man have demonstrated that the anti-inflammatory action of tolmetin is not due to pituitary-adrenal stimulation. Tolmetin inhibits prostaglandin synthetase in vitro and lowers the plasma level of prostaglandin E in man. This reduction in prostaglandin synthesis may be responsible for the anti-inflammatory action. Tolmetin does not appear to alter the course of the underlying disease in man.

Pharmacokinetics

Absorption

In patients with rheumatoid arthritis and in normal volunteers, tolmetin sodium is rapidly and almost completely absorbed with peak plasma levels being reached within 30-60 minutes after an oral therapeutic dose.

Distribution

In controlled studies, the time to reach peak tolmetin plasma concentration is approximately 20 minutes longer following administration of a 600 mg tablet, compared to an equivalent dose given as 200 mg tablets. The clinical meaningfulness of this finding, if any, is unknown. Tolmetin displays biphasic elimination from the plasma consisting of a rapid phase with a half-life of 1 to 2 hours followed by a slower phase with a half-life of about 5 hours. Peak plasma levels of approximately 40 µg/mL are obtained with a 400 mg oral dose.

Metabolism & Elimination

Essentially the entire administered dose is recovered in the urine in 24 hours either as an inactive oxidative metabolite or as conjugates of tolmetin. An 18-day multiple dose study demonstrated no accumulation of tolmetin when compared with a single dose.

In two fecal blood loss studies of 4 to 6 days duration involving 15 subjects each, tolmetin did not induce an increase in blood loss over that observed during a 4-day drug-free control period. In the same studies, aspirin produced a greater blood loss than occurred during the drug-free control period, and a greater blood loss than occurred during the tolmetin treatment period. In one of the two studies, indomethacin produced a greater fecal blood loss than occurred during the drug-free control period; in the second study, indomethacin did not induce a significant increase in blood loss.

Drug Interactions

ACE-inhibitors

NSAIDs may diminish the antihypertensive effect of ACE-inhibitors. This interaction should be given consideration in patients taking NSAIDs concomitantly with ACE-inhibitors.

Aspirin

As with other NSAIDs, concomitant administration of tolmetin sodium and aspirin is not generally recommended because of the potential of increased adverse effects.

Diuretics

NSAIDs can reduce the natriuretic effect of furosemide and thiazides in some patients. This response has been attributed to inhibition of renal prostaglandin synthesis. During concomitant therapy with NSAIDs, the patient should be observed closely for signs of renal failure, as well as to assure diuretic efficacy.

Lithium

NSAIDs have produced an elevation of plasma lithium levels and a reduction in renal lithium clearance. The mean minimum lithium concentration increased 15% and the renal clearance was decreased by approximately 20%. These effects have been attributed to inhibition of renal prostaglandin synthesis by the NSAIDs. Thus, when NSAIDs and lithium are administered concurrently, subjects should be observed carefully for signs of lithium toxicity.

Methotrexate

NSAIDs have been reported to competitively inhibit methotrexate accumulation in rabbit kidney slices. This may indicate that they could enhance the toxicity of methotrexate. Caution should be used when NSAIDs are administered concomitantly with methotrexate.

Warfarin

The effects of warfarin and NSAIDs on GI bleeding are synergistic, such that users of both drugs together have a risk of serious GI bleeding higher than users of either drug alone.

The in vitro binding of warfarin to human plasma proteins is unaffected by tolmetin, and tolmetin does not alter the prothrombin time of normal volunteers. However, increased prothrombin time and bleeding have been reported in patients on concomitant tolmetin and warfarin therapy.

Therefore, caution should be exercised when administering tolmetin to patients on anticoagulants.

Hypoglycemic Agents

In adult diabetic patients under treatment with either sulfonylureas or insulin there is no change in the clinical effects of either tolmetin or the hypoglycemic agents.

Drug / Laboratory Test Interactions

The metabolites of tolmetin sodium in urine have been found to give positive tests for proteinuria using tests which rely on acid precipitation as their endpoint (e.g., sulfosalicylic acid). No interference is seen in the tests for proteinuria using dye-impregnated commercially available reagent strips.

Drug-Food Interactions

In a controlled single-dose study, administration of tolmetin with milk had no effect on peak plasma tolmetin concentrations, but decreased total tolmetin bioavailability by 16%. When tolmetin was taken immediately after a meal, peak plasma tolmetin concentrations were reduced by 50% while total bioavailability was again decreased by 16%.

Adverse Drug Reaction

Headache, asthenia, chest pain, elevated blood pressure, edema, dizziness, drowsiness, depression, weight gain, weight loss, skin irritation, tinnitus, visual disturbance, small and transient decreases in hemoglobin and hematocrit not associated with gastrointestinal bleeding have occurred. These are similar to changes reported with other nonsteroidal anti-inflammatory drugs, urinary tract infection

Contraindication

Tolmetin is contraindicated in patients with known hypersensitivity to tolmetin sodium.

Tolmetin should not be given to patients who have experienced asthma, urticaria or allergic-type reactions after taking aspirin or other NSAIDs. Severe, rarely fatal, anaphylactic-like reactions to NSAIDs have been reported in such patients.

Tolmetin is contraindicated for the treatment of pre-operative pain in the setting of coronary artery bypass graft (CABG) surgery.

Dosage and Administration

For the relief of rheumatoid arthritis or osteoarthritis, the recommended starting dose for adults is 400 mg three times daily (1200 mg daily), preferably including a dose on arising and a dose at bedtime. To achieve optimal therapeutic effect the dose should be adjusted according to the patient's response after one or two weeks. Control is usually achieved at doses of 600-1800 mg daily in divided doses (generally t.i.d.). Doses larger than 1800 mg/day have not been studied and are not recommended.

For the relief of juvenile rheumatoid arthritis, the recommended starting dose for pediatric patients (2 years and older) is 20 mg/kg/day in divided doses (t.i.d. or q.i.d.). When control has been achieved, the usual dose ranges from 15 to 30 mg/kg/day. Doses higher than 30 mg/kg/day have not been studied, and, therefore, are not recommended.

Clinical Efficacy

Patients should be informed of the following information before initiating therapy with an NSAIDs and periodically during the course of ongoing therapy. Patients should also be encouraged to read the NSAID Medication guide that accompanies each prescription dispensed.

Tolmetin, like other NSAIDs, may cause serious cardiovascular side effects, such as myocardial infarction or stroke, which may result in hospitalization and even death. Although serious cardiorascular events can occur without warning symptoms, patients should be alert for the signs and symptoms of chest pain, shortness of breath, weakness, slurring of speech, and should ask for medical advice when observing any indicative signs or symptoms.

Tolmetin, like other NSAIDs, can cause GI discomfort and, rarely, serious GI side effects, such as ulcers and bleeding, which may result in hospitalization and even death. Although serious GI tract ulcerations and bleeding can occur without warning symptoms, patients should be alert for the signs and symptoms of ulcerations and bleeding, and should ask for medical advice when observing any indicative signs or symptoms including epigastric pain, dyspepsia, melena, and hematemesis Patients should be apprised of the importance of this follow-up.

Tolmetin, like other NSAIDs, can cause serious skin side effects such as exfoliative dermatitis, SJS, and TEN, which may result in hospitalizations and even death. Although serious skin reactions may occur without warning, patients should be alert for the signs and symptoms of skin rash and blisters, fever, or other signs of hypersensitivity, such as itching, and should ask for medical advice when observing any indicative signs or symptoms. Patients should be advised to stop the drug immediately if they develop any type of rash and contact their physicians as soon as possible.

Patients should promptly report signs or symptoms of unexplained weight gain or edema to their physicians.

Patients should be informed of the warning signs and symptoms of hepatotoxicity (e.g., nausea, fatigue, lethargy, pruritus, jaundice, right upper quadrant tenderness, and "flu-like" symptoms). If these occur, patients should be instructed to stop therapy and seek immediate medical therapy.

Patients should be informed of the signs of an anaphylactoid reaction (e.g., difficulty breathing, swelling of the face or throat). If these occur, patients should be instructed to seek immediate emergency help

In late pregnancy, as with other NSAIDs, tolmetin should be avoided because it may cause premature closure of the ductus arteriosus.

Pregnancy

Teratogenic Effects : Pregnancy Category C

Reproduction studies in rats and rabbits at doses up to 50 mg/kg (1.5 times the maximum clinical dose based on a body weight of 60 kg) revealed no evidence of teratogenesis or impaired fertility due to tolmetin. However, animal reproduction studies are not always predictive of human response. There are no adequate and well-controlled studies in pregnant women. Tolmetin should be used in pregnancy only if the potential benefit justifies the potential risk to the fetus.

Nonteratogenic Effects

Because of the known effects of NSAIDs on the fetal cardiovascular system (closure of ductus arteriosus), use during pregnancy (particularly late pregnancy) should be avoided.

Labor and Delivery

In rat studies with NSAIDs, as with other drugs known to inhibit prostaglandin synthesis, an increased incidence of dystocia, delayed parturition, and decreased pup survival occurred. The effects of tolmetin on labor and delivery in pregnant women are unknown.

Nursing Mothers

Tolmetin sodium has been shown to be secreted in human milk. Because of the potential for serious adverse reactions in nursing infants from tolmetin sodium, a decision should be made whether to discontinue nursing or to discontinue the drug, taking into account the importance of the drug to the mother.

Pediatric Use

Safety and effectiveness in pediatric patients below the age of 2 years have not been established.

General Precautions

Tolmetin cannot be expected to substitute for corticosteroids or to treat corticosteroid insufficiency. Abrupt discontinuation of corticosteroids may lead to disease exacerbation. Patients on prolonged corticosteroid therapy should have their therapy tapered slowly if a decision is made to discontinue corticosteroids.

The pharmacological activity of tolmetin in reducing fever and inflammation may diminish the utility of these diagnostic signs in detecting complications of presumed noninfectious, painful conditions.

Ophthalmological Effects

Because of ocular changes observed in animals and of reports of adverse eye findings with NSAIDs, it is recommended that patients who develop visual disturbances during treatment with tolmetin have ophthalmologic evaluations.

Hepatic Effects

Borderline elevations of one or more liver tests may occur in up to 15% of patients taking NSAIDs, including tolmetin. These laboratory abnormalities may progress, may remain unchanged, or may be transient with continuing therapy. Notable elevations of ALT or AST (approximately three or more times the upper limit of normal) have been reported in approximately 1% of patients in clinical trials with NSAIDs. In addition, rare cases of severe hepatic reactions, including jaundice and fatal fulminant hepatitis, liver necrosis, and hepatic failure, some of them with fatal outcomes have been reported.

A patient with symptoms and/or signs suggesting liver dysfunction, or in whom an abnormal liver test has occurred should be evaluated for evidence of the development of a more severe hepatic reaction while on therapy with tolmetin. If clinical signs and symptoms consistent with liver disease develop, or if systemic manifestations occur (e.g., eosinophilia, rash, etc.), tolmetin should be discontinued.

Hematological Effects

Anemia is sometimes seen in patients receiving NSAIDs, including tolmetin. This may be due to fluid retention, occult or gross GI blood loss, or an incompletely described effect upon erythropoiesis. Patients on long-term treatment with NSAIDs, including tolmetin, should have their hemoglobin or hematocrit checked if they exhibit any signs or symptoms of anemia. NSAIDs inhibit platelet aggregation and have been shown to prolong bleeding time in some patients. Unlike aspirin, their effect on platelet function is quantitatively less, of shorter duration, and reversible. Patients receiving tolmetin who may be adversely affected by alterations in platelet function, such as those with coagulation disorders or patients receiving anticoagulants, should be carefully monitored.

Preexisting Asthma

Patients with asthma may have aspirin-sensitive asthma. The use of aspirin in patients with aspirin-sensitive asthma has been associated with severe bronchospasm which can be fatal. Since cross reactivity, including bronchospasm, between aspirin and other NSAIDs has been reported in such aspirin-sensitive patients, tolmetin should not be administered to patients with this form of aspirin sensitivity and should be used with caution in patients with preexisting asthma.

Therapeutic Uses

Tolmetin is effective in treating both the acute flares and in the long-term management of the symptoms of rheumatoid arthritis, osteoarthritis and juvenile rheumatoid arthritis.

Rheumatoid arthritis or osteoarthritis

In patients with either rheumatoid arthritis or osteoarthritis, Tolmetin is as effective as aspirin and indomethacin in controlling disease activity, but the frequency of the milder gastrointestinal adverse effects and tinnitus was less than in aspirin-treated patients, and the incidence of central nervous system adverse effects was less than in indomethacin-treated patients.

Juvenile rheumatoid arthritis

In patients with juvenile rheumatoid arthritis, tolmetin is as effective as aspirin in controlling disease activity, with a similar incidence of adverse reactions. Mean SGOT values, initially elevated in patients on previous aspirin therapy, remained elevated in the aspirin group and decreased in the tolmetin group.

Brand Names

In India : Tolectin, Tolectin DS, Tolectin 600

In USA : Tolectin, Tolectin DS, Tolectin 600

In Other Countries:

Australia : Tolectin

Canada : Tolectin

Denmark : Tolectin

Italy : Tolectin

Mexico : Tolectin

South Africa : Tolectin

Spain : Artrocaptin

U.K : Tolectin

Zomepirac

History

Zomepirac is benzoyl pyrrole acetic acid derivative which is chemically closely related to the non-steroical anti-inflammatory agents. It is a potent analgesic with a predominantly peripheral action mediated through prostaglandin synthetase inhibition.

Description

Chemical Name : sodium salt of 1, 4-dimethyl – 5-(p-chlo-robenzoyl)-1H-pyrrole-2-acetic acid.

Appearance, Colour, Odor : Zomepirac is marketed as the sodium salt dehydrates; a pale yellow crystalline, odorless powder. Free acid appears as white, odorless crystalline powder.

Chemical structure

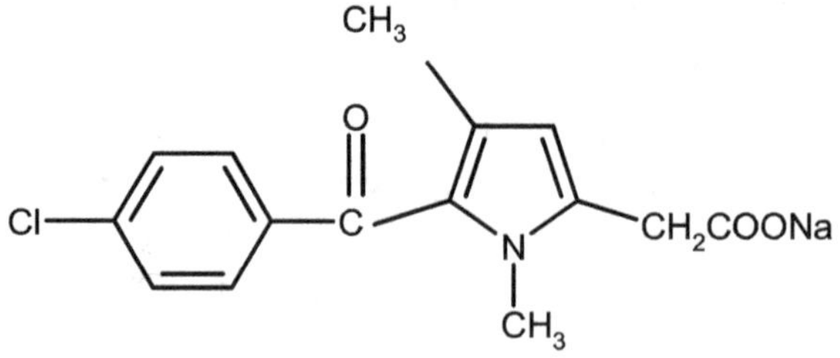

Molecular Weight - 313.56

Chemical formula - $C_{15}H_{13}ClNNaO_3$

Melting characteristics

Zomepirac can be conveniently crystallized from isopropanol. The crystalline product needle melts and decomposes at 178-179 °C. The sodium salt of zomepirac crystallizes as dehydrate from an isopropanol/water mixture. The salt melts at 295-296°C.

Solubility

Zomepirac is freely soluble in methanol, ethanol and hot isopropanol. It is soluble in acetone and chloroform, slightly soluble in ether and practically insoluble in methylene chloride, toluene and hydrocarbon solvents.

Pharmacokinetics

Because of its lipophilicity, zomepirac may owe at least part of its analgesic activity to an increased ability to penetrate into the spinal cord and brain and subsequently to the inhibition of prostaglandin synthesis within the central nervous system.

Absorption

On the basis of urinary recovery data, zomepirac is almost absorbed after oral administration of dosages of 25-200 mg to healthy subjects. Mean peak plasma concentrations of 2.47, 4.42 and 7.94 µg/ml were attained 44, 57 and 80 min after a single oral dose of 50, 100 or 200 mg, respectively. Bioavailability of zomepirac is the same after ingestion of tablets, capsules or an aqueous solution. Zomepirac is extensively bound to plasma albumin (98.5%) in man. Maximal plasma concentrations (4000 ng/ml) are reached in 1hour at dose of 100mg.)

Distribution

Tissue concentrations of radio labelled zomepirac in rats are in the stomach, kidneys, intestine, and liver, 2.9, 2.2, 1.7, and 0.5 times, respectively, plasma concentration 6 hours after oral administration of a 6mg / kg dose. The rat plasma concentrations of zomepirac and metabolites are about 55 times the tissue concentrations of highly perfused organs such as the heart and lungs, and about 50 times that of the brain. After 48 hours about 0.3% of the dose remains in the carcass of the rat, 0.1% of the dose being concentrated in the liver. Zomepirac is detected in the cerebrospinal fluid of cats 10 minutes after intravenous administrations were approximately 7% of plasma concentrations 24 hours after dosing.

Elimination

The elimination half-life of zomepirac is about 4 hours following a single dose, but may be increased following multiple doses. Plasma clearance after doses of 40mg/ kg in rhesus monkeys is depressed to less than one half that observed after doses of 5 and 10 mg/kg.

Zomepirac is excreted almost exclusively in the urine, the major metabolite being the glucuronide conjugate, which accounts for about 57% of radioactivity after a 25 mg dose. Hydroxyzomepirac and 4-chlorobenzoic acid are minor metabolites and they are approximately 200-300 times less active than zomepirac as inhibitors of human platelet aggregation *in vitro*. About 22% of the dose is excreted in urine unchanged.

Carprofen

Description

It is a white, crystalline compound. The relative anti-inflammatory activity of carprofen is approximately: carprofen $\approx$ indomethacin, piroxicam, diclofenac > phenylbutazone > ibuprofen > aspirin analgesic and antipyretic activities have also been shown to be similar to indomethacin and greater than phenylbutazone or aspirin. Carprofen is reported to be 16 times less active than indomethacin in producing gastric ulcers in mice. Carprofen causes significantly less platelet aggregation inhibition than aspirin does; carprofen does not alter buccal mucosal bleeding time in healthy dogs when administered at recommended dosages.

Chemical group: Aryl-propionic acid class of non-steroidal anti-inflammatory drug.

Chemical name : (±)-6-Chloro-alpha-methylcarbazole-2-acetic acid.

Molecular formula : $C_{15}H_{12}ClNO_2$.

NH

COOH

CH$_3$

Cl   Carprofen

Molecular weight : 273.72.

Solubility : Freely soluble in ethanol, but practically insoluble in water at 25 °C.

Chirality : Carprofen contains an asymmetrical carbon atom and exists in two enantiomeric forms. Differences in pharmacokinetics and pharmacodynamics between the two enantiomers occur in animals and can also vary significantly among species. Currently, commercially available products contain a racemic (50:50) mixture of the two enantiomers, S(+) and R(–).

Pharmacodynamic

The mechanisms of action of carprofen are not completely understood. This lack of clarity may be due to species differences, to differing methodologies in the studies performed, and to the evolving understanding of anti-inflammatory activity and tests for measuring it. Inhibition of cyclooxygenase is believed to be the mechanism of action for the anti-inflammatory effect of carprofen.

Carprofen has been shown to inhibit the release of prostagladins from rat polymorphonuclear leucocytes, an acute inflammatory reaction, and human rheumatoid synovial cells, a chronic inflammatory reaction.

Pharmacokinetic

Absorption

Oral : Carprofen is rapidly and almost completely absorbed; greater than 90% bioavailability.

Subcutaneous : When administered subcutaneously at a dose of about 2 mg per kg of body weight (mg/kg), carprofen has a slower rate of absorption than when administered orally. But total drug absorption in the first 12 hours after a single dose and at steady state with repeated doses is similar for the two routes of administration.

Distribution

Racemic form does not appear to affect transfer from plasma to transudate or exudate, as demonstrated in calves and dogs; the R(–)-enantiomer continues to predominate. In dogs and horses, concentration of carprofen was greater in transudate and exudate in tissue cages or pouches than in plasma twenty-four to forty-eight hours after administration. However, penetration into transudate is limited until inflammation is present. Penetration of carprofen into the synovial fluid of healthy joints of horses is also limited but is expected to be significantly higher with inflammation.

Metabolites

70 to 80% of carprofen metabolites are eliminated in the feces and 10 to 20% in the urine. Identified metabolites include an ester glucuronide and ether glucuronides of 2 phenolic metabolites, 7-hydroxy carprofen and 8-hydroxy carprofen. Some enterohepatic circulation of the S (+)-enantiomer metabolites occurs; about 34% of the dose is recirculated.

Adverse Drug Reaction

Lactation

Carprofen has limited distribution into milk in healthy animals. With a single low intravenous dose (0.7 mg/kg), concentration in milk has been reported to be less than 0.02 mcg/mL of milk and, with five daily doses, concentrations increased to only 0.03 mcg/mL.

Gastrointestinal effects

Vomiting, diarrhea, constipation, inappetence, melena, hematemesis, gastrointestinal ulceration, gastrointestinal bleeding, pancreatitis, hepatic effects (inappetence, vomiting, jaundice, acute hepatic toxicity, hepatic enzyme elevation, abnormal liver function tests, hyper bilirubinemia, bilirubinuria, hypo albuminemia).

Neurologic effects

Ataxia, paresis, paralysis, seizures, vestibular signs, disorientation.

Urinary effects

Hematuria, polyuria, polydipsia, urinary incontinence, urinary tract infection, azotemia, acute renal failure, tubular abnormalities, including acute tubular necrosis, renal tubular necrosis, glucosuria.

Behavioral effects

Sedation, lethargy, hyperactivity, restlessness, aggressiveness.

Hematologic effects

Immune-mediated hemolytic anemia, immune-mediated thrombocytopenia, blood loss anemia, epistaxis.

Dermatologic effects

Pruritis, increased shedding, alopecia, pyotraumatic moist dermatitis, necrotizing panniculitis/vasculitis, ventral ecchymosis.

Immunologic effects or hypersensitivity

Facial swelling, hives, erythema.

Clinical Efficacy

Pain (treatment) **:** Although the safety and efficacy have not been established, there is evidence to suggest that oral or parenteral carprofen can be effective in the treatment of pain and inflammation.

Clinical effects of overdose

The following effects have been selected on the basis of their potential clinical significance (possible signs in parentheses where appropriate)—not necessarily inclusive

Dose

Usual dose : Inflammation, musculoskeletal; or Pain, musculoskeletal—Dogs: Oral, 4.4 mg per kg of body weight every twenty-four hours or 2.2 mg per kg of body weight every twelve hours Pain.

Therapeutic Uses

Inflammation, musculoskeletal (treatment); or Pain.

Ketorolac

Description

It is a novel NSAIDs with potent analgesic and modest anti-inflammatory activity. In postoperative pain it has equaled the efficacy of morphine, but does not interact with opoid receptors and is free of respiratory depressant, producing hypotensive and constipating side effect. It inhibits PG synthesis and is believed to relieve pain by peripheral mechanisms, it has compared favorably with aspirin. Platelet aggregration is inhibited for short periods.

Ketorolac is a potent analgesic but only a moderately effective anti-inflammatory drug. It is one of the few NSAIDs approved for parenteral administration. It is categorized under pyrrolo-pyrrole derivative.

Ketorolac contains not less then 98.5% and not more then 101.5% of $C_{15}H_{13}NO_3$ calculated on the dried basis.

It is a white to off-white, crystalline powder.freely soluble in the water and in methyl alcohol: slightly soluble in alcohol in dehydrated alcohol, in acetone, in acetonitrile, in butyl alcohol, in dichloromethane, in dioxan, in ethyl acetate, in hexane, and toluene. pH of a 1% solution in water is between 5.7 and 6.7. Store in airtight containers and protect from light.

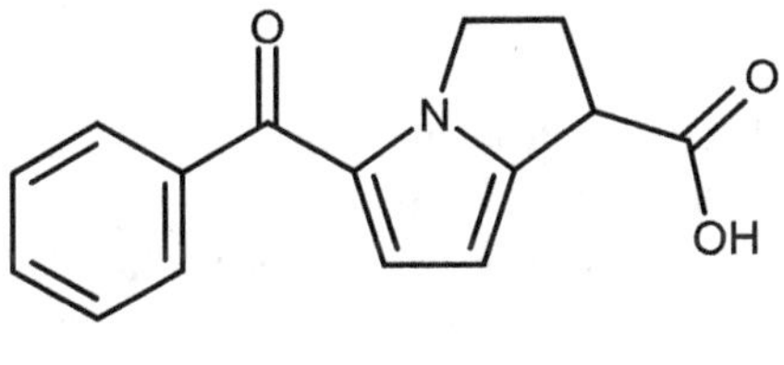

IUPAC Name (±)-5-benzoyl-2, 3-dihydro-1$\underline{H}$-pyrrolizine-1-carboxylic acid, 2-amino- 2-(hydroxymethyl)-1,3-propanediol.

Formula - $C_{15}H_{13}NO_3$

Mol weight - 376.4 g/mol

Ketorolac, like other 2-arylpropionate derivatives contains a chiral carbon in the β-position of the propionate moiety. As such there are two possible enantiomers of ketorolac with the potential for different biological effects and metabolism for each enantiomer.

Pharmacodynamics

Mechanism of action

The primary mechanism of action responsible for ketorolac is anti-inflammatory/antipyretic/analgesic effects is the inhibition of prostaglandin synthesis by competitive blocking of the enzyme cyclooxygenase (COX). Like most NSAIDs, ketorolac is a non-selective cyclooxygenase inhibitor.

As with other NSAIDs, the mechanism of the drug is associated with the chiral S form. Conversion of the R enantiomer into the S enantiomer has been shown to occur in the metabolism of ibuprofen; it is unknown whether it occurs in the metabolism of ketorolac. Its goes a phase 3 reactions.

Pharmacokinetics

Absorption

Ketorolac is rapidly absorbed whether given orally or intramuscularly, achieving peak plasma concentration in 30 to 50 minutes.

Distribution

Oral bioavailability is about 80%. Almost totally bound to plasma proteins.

Metabolism

The major metabolic pathway is glucuronidation.$T_{1/2}$ -- 5-7hr.

The major metabolites are the acyl gluronide and p- hydroxyketorolac, which represent 77% and 12% respectively.

Excreation

It is excreted with an elimination half-life of 4 to 6 hours. Urinary excretion accounts for about 90% of eliminated drug, with about 60% excreted unchanged and the remainder as a glucuronidated conjugate. The rate of elimination is reduced in the elderly and in patients with renal failure.

Drug Interactions

Ketorolac is highly bound to human plasma protein (mean 99.2%).

Warfarin, Digoxin, Salicylate, and Heparin

The *in vitro* binding of warfarin to plasma proteins is only slightly reduced by ketorolac, when ketorolac plasma concentrations reach 5 to10 mg/mL. Ketorolac does not alter digoxin protein binding. In vitro studies indicate that, at therapeutic concentrations of salicylate (300 mg/mL), the binding of ketorolac was reduced from approximately 99.2% to 97.5%; representing a potential two fold increase in unbound ketorolac plasma levels. Therapeutic concentrations of digoxin, warfarin, ibuprofen, naproxen, piroxicam, acetaminophen, phenytoin and tolbutamide did not alter ketorolac protein binding.

Ketorolac should not be given to patients already receiving anticoagulants or to those who will require prophylactic anticogulant therapy. Including low dose heparin. The risk of ketorolac-associated bleeding is increased by other NSAIDs or aspirin and by oxypentifylline and concomitant use should be avoided. Probenecid increases the half-life and plasma concentration of ketorolac and the two drugs should not be given together.

Adverse Drug Reactions

1. **General** Edema. Less frequently, hypersensitivity reactions (such as anaphylaxis, bronchospasm, laryngeal edema, tongue edema, hypotension), flushing, weight gain, or fever. Very infrequently, asthenia.

2. **Cardiovascular** Hypertension. Less frequently, palpitation, pallor, or syncope.

3. **Dermatologic** Rash or pruritus. Less frequently, Lyell's syndrome, Stevens-Johnson syndrome, musculo-papular rash, exfoliative dermatitis, or urticaria.

4. **Gastrointestinal** Nausea, dyspepsia, gastrointestinal pain, constipation, diarrhea, flatulence, gastrointestinal fullness, vomiting or stomatitis. Less frequently, peptic ulceration, gastrointestinal hemorrhages, gastrointestinal perforation, rectal bleeding, gastritis, anorexia, or increased appetite.

5. **Hemic and lymphatic** Purpura. Less frequently, postoperative wound hemorrhage, thrombocytopenia, epistaxis, or anemia. Very infrequently, leukopenia or eosinophilia.

6. **Neurological** Drowsiness, dizziness, headache, sweating, injection site pain. Less frequently convulsions, vertigo, tremors, abnormal

dreams, hallucinations, or euphoria. Very infrequently, paresthesia, depression, insomnia, inability to concentrate, nervousness, excessive thirst, dries mouth, abnormal thinking, hyperkinesis, or stupor.

7. **Respiratory** Less frequently, dyspnea, asthma and pulmonary edema. Very infrequently, rhinitis or cough.

8. **Urogenital** Less frequently, acute renal failure. Very infrequently polyuria or increased urinary frequency.

Dose and Administration

Orally: 10 to 20 mg every 4 to 6 h (6 to 8 for the elderly) with a maximum of 40mg daily. Intravenously; intial does of 10mg followed by 10 to 30 mg every 4 to 6 h. Maximum daily dose is to 90mg and 60mg for the elderly and patients weighing less than 50kg. Ketorolac administrated intramuscularly (Im), intravenously (IV), orally.

Clinical Efficacy

Ketorolac is a non-steroidal agent with potent analgesic and moderate anti-inflammatory activity. It is administered as the tromethamine salt orally, intramuscularly, intravenously and as a topical ophthalmic solution. Clinical studies indicate single dose efficacy to be greater than that of morphine, pethidine and pentazocine in moderate to severe operative pain with some evidence of a more favorable adverse effect profile than morphine or pethidine. In single dose studies, ketorolac has also compared favorably with aspirin, paracetamol and other non-steroidal anti-inflammatory drugs (NSAIDs). It also has exhibited anti-pyretic activity in rats. Like other NSAIDs, ketorolac is an inhibitor of prostaglandin synthesis. As it possesses potent analgesic and moderate anti-inflammatory activity, its use has an advantage over using a combination of two drugs with individual antinflammatory and analgesic properties for post-operative analgesia.

Therapeutic Uses

Ketorolac (administered as the tromethamine salt,) is used for postoperative pain, as an alternative to opioid agents, and is administered intramuscularly or orally. Typical intramuscularly doses are 30 to 90 mg, and oral doses are 5 to 30 mg. Ketorolac probably should not be used for obstetric analgesia. Oral ketorolac has been used for treatment of chronic pain states, for which it appears to be superior to aspirin. Topical ketorolac may be useful for inflammatory conditions in the eye and is approved for the treatment of seasonal allergic conjunctivitis. Ketorolac is also used as 0.5 % eye drops to relieve itching associated with seasonal allergic conjunctitis.

Brand names

Ketorol, Zorovon, Ketanov, Torolac

Tromethamine

Description

A white crystalline powder or colorless crystals

Synonyms THAM : Tri hydroxy methamino methane, TRIS: Tris (hydroxymethyl) aminomethane

IUPAC name 2-Amino-2-hydroxymethyl-1, 3-propanediol

Molecular Formula – $C_2H_{11}NO_3$

Mol Weight - 121

Chemistry

A crystalline compound with a melting point of 171-172°C; soluble in water, ethylene glycol, methanol, and ethanol; used to make surface-active agents, vulcanization accelerators, and pharmaceuticals, and as a titrimetric standard.

Also known as THAM; trimethylol aminomethane; TRIS; trisaminetri-sbuffers

Pharmacodynamics

Mechanisms of action

Inhibition of prostaglandin synthesis by competitive blocking of the enzyme cyclooxygenase (COX).

Pharmacokinetics

Tromethamine is an alkalinizing agent, which acts as a proton (hydrogen ion) acceptor. Tromethamine is a weak base; it attracts and combines with hydrogen ions and their associated acid anions and the resulting salts are excreted in urine. Tromethamine can combine with lactic, pyruvic, and other metabolic acids and with carbonic acid. The reaction of tromethamine with acid is represented as follows:

Absorption

It is absorbed by orally or intravenous route.

Distribution

At pH 7.4, approximately 70% of the tromethamine present in plasma is in the ionized (protonated) form; if pH is decreased from pH 7.4, the ionized fraction of the drug is increased. In contrast to the ionized fraction of tromethamine, which upon administration reacts only with acid in the extracellular fluids, the fraction of the dose, which remains un-ionized at physiologic pH, is thought to be capable of penetrating the cell membrane to combine with intracellular acid.

Metabolism and Elimination

Ionized tromethamine (chiefly as the bicarbonate salt) is rapidly and preferentially excreted in urine at a rate that depends on the infusion rate. Transient decreases in blood glucose concentration may occur during administration of tromethamine. When larger than recommended doses are used or when administration is too rapid, hypoglycemia may persist for several hours after the drug is discontinued.

Drug Interaction

Local reactions associated with administration of tromethamine may include local irritation and tissue inflammation or infection at the site of injection, a febrile respose, chemical phlebitis, venospasm, and thrombosis.

Adverse Drug Reaction

It produces local irritation, respiratory acidosis and respiratory depression. Local reactions associated with administration of tromethamine may include local irritation and tissue inflammation or infection at the site of injection, a febrile respose, chemical phlebitis, venospasm, and thrombosis. The drug should be administered through a large needle or indwelling catheter to minimize venous irritation by the highly alkaline tromethamine solution. Extravasation may result in inflammation, necrosis, and sloughing of overlying skin. If perivascular infiltration occurs, tromethamine administration should be discontinued immediately. Infiltration of the affected area with 1% procaine hydrochloride, to which hyaluronidase has been added, will often reduce venospasm and also will dilute any tromethamine remaining in the tissues locally. Local infiltration of α-adrenergic blocking agent, such as phentolamine mesylate, into the vasospastic area has been recommended. If necessary, nerve block of autonomic fibers to the affected area may be performed.

Respiratory depression may occur in patients receiving tromethamine, especially in those with chronic hypoventilation or in those receiving other drugs that depress respiration.

It produces gastrointestinal disturbances including gastrointestinal bleeding (especially in the elderly) and peptic ulceration. Hypersensitivity reaction such as anaphylaxis, rash, brochospasm, laryngeal edema, and hypotension have also occurred. Other adverse effects are drowsiness, dizziness, mental and sensory changes, psychotic reaction, sweating, dry mouth, thirst, fever, convulsions, myalgia, aseptic meningitis, dyspnoea, pulmonary edema, bradycardia, chest pain and palpitations.

Dosages and Administration

Dosage of tromethamine depends on the severity and progression of the acidosis. Determinations of blood pH, carbon dioxide tension, and bicarbonate, glucose, and electrolyte concentrations should be performed before, during, and following administration of the drug.

Clinical Efficacy

The safety and efficacy of tromethamine in pediatric patients is based on extensive (over 30 years) clinical experience documented in the medical literature and by safety surveillance. Tromethamine has been used in the treatment of severe cases of metabolic acidosis with concurrent respiratory acidosis in neonates and infants with respiratory failure, because unlike sodium bicarbonate, tromethamine does not elevate carbon dioxide tension ($PaCO_2$). The drug also has been used in neonates and infants with hypernatremia and metabolic acidosis to avoid the additional sodium given with the bicarbonate. However, because the osmotic effects of tromethamine are greater and large continuous doses of the drug are required, sodium bicarbonate is preferred to tromethamine in the treatment of acidosis in neonates and infants with respiratory distress syndrome (RDS).

IV infusions of tromethamine via low-lying umbilical venous catheters have been associated with incidences of hepatocellular necrosis. In addition, hypoglycemia may occur when tromethamine is used in premature and even in full-term neonates. Tromethamine is contraindicated in neonates with chronic respiratory acidosis and salicylate intoxication.

Therapeutic Uses

Tromethamine is an organic amine proton acceptor, which is used as an alkalinizing agent in the treatment of metabolic acidosis. It also acts as osmotic diuretic. Tromethamine is used for the prevention and correction of metabolic acidosis associated with cardiac bypass surgery.

Although tromethamine may also be used as an alkalinizing agent in cardiac arrest, there are few data indicating that therapy with buffers improves the outcome in cardiac arrest. However, therapy with an alkalinizing agent may be beneficial in some patients but generally should be used only after more proven methods for advanced cardiovascular life support (ACLS) such as defibrillation, cardiac compression, support of ventillation including intubation, and vasopresssor therapy have been ineffective.

Tromethamine may also be used to titrate the excess acidity of stored blood (blood that has been preserved with anticoagulant citrate dextrose [ACD] solution) used to prime the pump-oxygenator during cardiac bypass surgery. The drug also has been used to treat metabolic acidosis associated with status asthmaticus and with the neonatal respiratory distress syndrome. If respiratory acidosis accompanies metabolic acidosis, ventilation must be maintained by artificial means; the drug is not recommended in patients with respiratory acidosis alone, since the drug may depress ventilation by decreasing carbon dioxide tension.

Mefenamic Acid

Descrpition

Mefenamic acid is in a class of drugs called nonsteroidal anti-inflammatory drugs (NSAIDs). Mefenamic acid works by reducing hormones that cause inflammation and pain in the body. Mefenamic acid is used to reduce pain caused by various conditions including menstruation.

Synonyms

Acide Mefenamique, Bafameritin-M, Bafhameritin-M, Bonabol, Coslan

Molecular formula : $C_{15}H_{15}NO_2$

Molecular weight : -241.3

Structural formula

Solubility : sparingly soluble in ether and soluble in ethanol (95%) and chloroform, practically soluble in water.

Pharmacokinetics

Absorption

Mefenamic acid is rapidly absorbed after oral administration. In two 500-mg single oral dose studies, the mean extent of absorption was 30.5 mcg/hr/mL (17% CV). The bioavailability of the capsule relative to an IV dose or an oral solution has not been studied.

The effect of food on the rate and extent of absorption of mefenamic acid has not been studied. Concomitant ingestion of antacids containing magnesium hydroxide has been shown to significantly increase the rate and extent of mefenamic acid absorption.

Distribution

Mefenamic acid has been reported as being greater than 90% bound to albumin. The relationship of unbound fraction to drug concentration has not been studied. The apparent volume of distribution (Vz_{ss}/F) estimated following a 500-mg oral dose of mefenamic acid was 1.06 L/kg. Based on its physical and chemical properties, mefenamic acid is expected to be excreted in human breast milk.

Metabolism

Mefenamic acid is metabolized by cytochrome P450 enzyme CYP2C9 to 3-hydroxymethyl mefenamic acid. Further oxidation to a 3-carboxymefenamic acid may occur. The activity of these metabolites has not been studied. The metabolites may undergo glucuronidation and mefenamic acid is also glucuronidated directly. A peak plasma level approximating 20 mcg/mL was observed at 3 hours for the hydroxy metabolite and its glucuronide (n=6) after a single 1-gram dose. Similarly, a peak plasma level of 8 mcg/mL was observed at 6-8 hours for the carboxy metabolite and its glucuronide.

Excretion

Approximately fifty-two percent of a mefenamic acid dose is excreted into the urine primarily as glucuronides of mefenamic acid (6%), 3-hydroxymefenamic acid (25%) and 3-carboxymefenamic acid (21%). The fecal route of elimination accounts for up to 20% of the dose, mainly in the form of unconjugated 3-carboxymefenamic acid.

The elimination half-life of mefenamic acid is approximately two hours. Half-lives of metabolites I and II have not been precisely reported, but appear to be longer than the parent compound. The metabolites may accumulate in patients with renal or hepatic failure. The mefenamic acid glucuronide may bind irreversibly to plasma proteins. Because both renal and hepatic excretion are significant pathways of elimination, dosage adjustments in patients with renal or hepatic dysfunction may be necessary.mefenamic acid should not be administered to patients with preexisting renal disease or in patients with significantly impaired renal function.

Adverse Effects

- Allergic reaction: Itching or hives, swelling in face or hands, swelling or tingling in mouth or throat, chest tightness, trouble breathing
- Blistering, peeling, red skin rash
- Bloody or black, tarry stools
- Change in quantity and frequency of urination
- Chest pain, shortness of breath, or coughing up blood
- Dark-colored urine or pale stools
- Flu-like symptoms
- Numbness or weakness in arm or leg, or on one side of body
- Pain in lower leg
- Problems with vision, speech, or walking
- Shortness of breath, cold sweat, and bluish-colored skin
- Sudden and severe stomach pain, nausea, vomiting, fever, and lightheadedness
- Sudden or severe headache
- Swelling in hands, ankles, or feet

Dosage and Administration

The dose and frequency should be adjusted to suit an individual patient's needs. For the relief of acute pain in adults and adolescents 14 years of age, the recommended dose is 500 mg as an initial dose followed by 250 mg every 6 hours as needed, usually not to exceed one week. Take Mefenamic acid with food if possible. If it upsets the stomach, be sure to take it with food or an antacid or with a full glass of milk. Take Mefenamic acid exactly as prescribed by doctor.

Therapeutic Uses

Mefenamic acid has analgesic, anti-inflammatory and anti-pyretic properties. It inhibits the synthesis of prostaglandins. Mefenamic acid shows central and peripheral action and it owes these properties to its capacity to inhibit cyclooxygenase.

Drug Interactions

Aspirin : As with other NSAIDs, concomitant administration of mefenamic acid and aspirin is not generally recommended because of the potential of increased adverse effects.

Methotrexate : NSAIDs have been reported to competitively inhibit methotrexate accumulation in rabbit kidney slices. This may indicate that they could enhance the toxicity of methotrexate. Caution should be used when NSAIDs are administered concomitantly with methotrexate.

ACE inhibitors : NSAIDs may diminish the antihypertensive effect of ACE inhibitors. This interaction should be given consideration in patients taking NSAIDs concomitantly with ACE inhibitors.

Furosemide : Clinical studies, as well as post-marketing observations, have shown that NSAIDs can reduce the natriuretic effect of furosemide and thiazides in some patients. This response has been attributed to inhibition of renal prostaglandin synthesis. During concomitant therapy of mefenamic acid with furosemide, the patient should be observed closely for signs of renal failure, as well as to assure diuretic efficacy.

Lithium : NSAIDs have produced an elevation of plasma lithium levels and a reduction in renal lithium clearance. The mean minimum lithium concentration increases 15% and the renal clearance decreases by approximately 20%. These effects have been attributed to inhibition of renal prostaglandin synthesis by the NSAID. Thus, when NSAIDs and lithium are administered concurrently, subjects should be observed carefully for signs of lithium toxicity.

Warfarin : The effects of warfarin and NSAIDs on GI bleeding are synergistic, such that users of both drugs together have a risk of serious GI bleeding higher than users of either drug alone.

Antacids : In a single dose study (n = 6), ingestion of an antacid containing 1.7-gram of magnesium hydroxide with 500-mg of mefenamic acid increased the Cmax and AUC of mefenamic acid by 125% and 36%, respectively.

A number of compounds are inhibitors of CYP2C9 including fluconazole, lovastatin and trimethoprim. Drug interaction studies of mefenamic acid and these compounds have not been conducted. The possibility of altered safety and efficacy should be considered when mefenamic acid is used concomitantly with these drugs.

Side Effects

Mefenamic acid is known to cause an upset stomach, therefore it is recommended to take prescribed doses together with food or milk. Instances of drowsiness may also occur. As such, it is recommended to avoid driving or consuming alcohol while taking this medication. Other known mild side effects of mefenamic acid include headaches, nervousness and vomiting. Serious side effects may include diarrhea, bloody vomit, blurred vision, skin rash, itching and swelling, sore throat and fever. It is advised to consult a doctor immediately if these symptoms appear while taking this medication.

Brand Names

In India : Ponstel

In USA : Postan

In Maxico : Postan 500

Flufenamic Acid

Description

Flufenamic acid is an anthranilic acid derivative with analgesic, anti-inflammatory, and antipyretic properties. It is used in musculoskeletal and joint disorders and administered by mouth and topically.

Molecular formula: $C_{14}H_{10}F_3NO_2$

Molecular weight : 281.23

Chemicalname : 2-{[3-(Trifluoromethyl) Phenyl] Amino} Benzoic Acid

Structural formula :

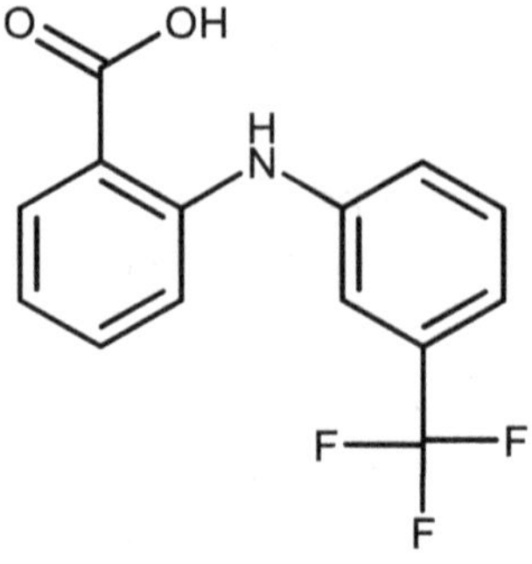

Solubility *:* Freely soluble in water (concentrated solutions are liable to deposit crystals of the hexahydrate) and in ethanol *(95%);* practically insoluble in ether.

Storage *:* Store in tightly-closed, light-resistant containers.

Pharmacodynamics

Flufenamic acid is a drug belongs to a class of NSAIDs (nonsteroidal anti-inflammatory drug) acts by inhibiting isoforms of cyclo-oxygenase 1 and 2. It has an activity to treat inflammatory rheumatoid diseases and relieve acute pain. It is effective against period pains, pain after surgery, and fever.

Drug Interaction

The effects of the non-steroidal anti-inflammatory drug (NSAIDs) flufenamic acid on H+ production in isolated and enriched guinea-pig parietal cells and on H+/K(+)-ATPase activity in ion-tight inside-out membrane vesicles from pig gastric mucosa were studied. At low concentrations (0.1 and 1.0 mumol/L), flufenamic acid increased the secretory response of parietal cells to dibutyryl cyclic AMP (dbcAMP). At higher concentrations (10 and 100 mumol/L) it progressively inhibited basal and dbcAMP-stimulated acid production. Flufenamic acid (10 mumol/L) increased K+ (0.5-10.0 mmol/L) and K+ (0.5-1.0 mmol/L) plus gramicidin-stimulated ATPase activity in gastric membrane vesicles. The Km value for K+ (1.6 and 1.0 mmol/L in the absence and presence of gramicidin, respectively) was decreased to 0.8 and 0.5 mmol/L, respectively. At higher concentrations (greater than or equal to 50 mumol/L), flufenamic acid inhibited K+ plus gramicidin-stimulated ATPase activity (inhibited concentration at 50% [IC50] = 186 mumol/L) and reduced the proton concentration (IC50 = 50 mumol/L). It is concluded that flufenamic acid-induced enhancement of dibutyryl cyclic AMP-stimulated H+ production in the parietal cell reflects the stimulation of H+/K(+)-ATPase.

Pirprofen

Description

Pirprofen is a non-steroidal anti-inflammatory drug, related structurally to drugs such as ibuprofen, ketoprofen and naproxen a nonsteroidal antiinflammatory drug (NSAIDs).

Synonyms - 3-Chloro-4-(3-pyrrolin-1-yl) hydratropic acid

Molecular formula - C_{14}-H_{14}-Cl NO_2

Molecular weight - 263.5

Chemical structure

Metabolism of pirprofen

Pirprofen was well absorbed by man, after oral administration of a solution of 14C-labeled compound. The major route of elimination of radioactivity in all four species was renal, mostly in the form of metabolites. Twelve metabolites of pirprofen, accounting for 80% or more of the urinary radioactivity, were identified in the urine of the four species. The metabolic pathways of pirprofen involved oxidation to the pyrrole analogue, and oxidation of the pyrroline double bond to an epoxide, followed by opening of the oxirane ring to a trans-diol derivative. Scission of the pyrroline or pyrrole ring was also observed, leading to the corresponding aniline type metabolite, part of which underwent subsequent acetylation. Conjugation of the propionic acid functionality with glucuronic acid was found to be extensive in the mouse, rhesus, and man, but not in the rat. Conjugation with taurine was also observed in the rat and mouse.

Dosage and administraction

Pirprofen was judged by doctors to be of good or excellent efficacy in 79% of patients, as compared to 24% on placebo. After 7 days, the results were confirmed with 63% of good and excellent efficacy in the pirprofen group versus 12% for the placebo (p less than 0,001). The two other studies compared pirprofen (800 mg/day) to ketoprofen (300 mg/day). One of the trials was conducted in a medical center for sports injuries on 79 patients. After 7 days of treatment, improvement was noted in 58 to 80% of the patients. The better results observed in sports medicine as compared to the traditional rheumatological a disease is due to the difference in the recruitment of the patients. In both trials, the 2 active drugs had a clear, comparable efficacy. Side effects were rare: primarily gastralgia which were more frequent amongst patients treated by pirprofen (11 out of 25) than that on placebo (4 out of 26). In trials comparing pirprofen and ketoprofen, side effects, especially gastralgia were noted in 30% of the patients in each group.

Therapeutic efficacy

Published clinical trials indicate that pirprofen 600 to 1200 mg/day as 2 or 3 divided doses is a suitable alternative to usual therapeutic dosages of aspirin, flurbiprofen, ibuprofen, indomethacin, ketoprofen, naproxen, piroxicam and sulindac in the treatment of rheumatoid arthritis, osteoarthritis, ankylosing spondylitis, musculoskeletal disorders and non-articular rheumatism. More studies are required to evaluate its potential relative to other commonly used drugs in the treatment of gout, juvenile rheumatoid arthritis and dysmenorrhoea. In patients with acute postsurgical, trauma or cancer pain, single oral or intramuscular doses of pirprofen 200 to 400 mg provide equivalent analgesic activity to usual therapeutic doses of aspirin, diflunisal, ketoprofen, noramidopyrine, paracetamol and pentazocine.

Side effects

At equivalent analgesic or anti-inflammatory dosages, pirprofen probably causes fewer side effects than aspirin and appears to be as well tolerated as the other agents with which it has been compared. Long term tolerability, particularly compared with some of the newer, purportedly less gastrotoxic agents or formulations, needs to be investigated further. Pirprofen does not appear likely to offer any particular advantage with respect to efficacy and tolerability over other non-steroidal anti-inflammatory drugs, except aspirin. However, as no one agent is the most suitable drug for all patients requiring such therapy, pirprofen may be considered along with other drugs of this type in the therapy of arthritic conditions and acute pain states.

US Brand Names

minizide

Fenbufen

Description

Fenbufen is a non-steroid anti-inflammatory drug which has also analgesic and antipyretic function. It inhibits synthesis of prostaglandinins. Administered orally it is easily absorbed from alimentary tract and then quickly metabolised into pharmacologically active compounds with effective half-time 10-11 hours. Fenbufen and its metabolites have strong bonds with serum proteins (over 99%).

Chemical name: fenbufenum 4 (biphenyl - 4 –yn) – 4 oxobutyric acid.

Molecular weight - 254.0943

Melting point -186°C to 189°C.

Pharmacodynamic

Fenbufen belongs to a group of medicines called non-steroidal anti-inflammatory drugs (NSAIDs). Fenbufen is converted in the liver to its active form. This then works by blocking the action of a substance in the body called cyclo-oxygenase. Cyclo-oxygenase is involved in the production of various chemicals in the body, some of which are known as prostaglandins. Prostaglandins are produced in response to injury or certain diseases and cause pain, swelling and inflammation. As fenbufen stops the production of prostaglandins, it relieves inflammation and pain. All the medicines in this group (NSAIDs) reduce inflammation caused by the body's own immune system and are effective pain killers.

Pharmacokinetic

Absorption

Fenbufen is rapidly absorbed from the gastroiintestinal tract to the extent of at least 78%. Food reduced the rate but not the extent of absorption. Peak serum concentrations of total drug related compounds were reached by 2 hr, at which time fenbufen accounted for only 11% of these substances. The remaining drug related material consisted of two metabolites: gamma-hydroxy (1,1'-biphenyl)-4-butanoic acid and (1,1'-biphenyl)-4-acetic acid. Steady state serum concentrations were reached within a week with multiple dosing regimens.

Distribution

Fenbufen is absorbed from the gastrointestinal tract and peak plasma concentration is reached in about 70 min. fenbufen is over 99% bound to plasma protein.

Metabolism and elimination

The ratio of fenbufen to its circulating metabolites did not change over a month of daily dosing. Only traces of fenbufen and metabolites were present in the cellular components of blood or in human milk, but significant amounts (concentrations one-third those in serum) were measured in the synovial fluid of arthritic patients. Fenbufen and its circulating metabolites were highly bound (> 98%) to human serum in vitro, but at therapeutic levels showed very small or no effects on the serum binding of various other commonly used drugs. Concomitant administration of fenbufen and acetylsalicylic acid (ASA) resulted in decreased serum concentration of fenbufen and its metabolites compared to those obtained from fenbufen administration alone. In addition to the serum metabolites, three more transformation products were identified in urine: 4'-hydroxy(1,1'-biphenyl)-4-acetic acid, gamma,4'-dihydroxy(1,1'-biphenyl)-4-butanoic acid and beta, gamma-dyhydroxy(1,1'-biphenyl)-4-butanoic acid. Fenbufen is metabolized in are reported to a plasma half life about and mainly eliminated as conjugated in the urine.

Drug Interaction

Fenbufen should not be taken with any other non-steroidal anti-inflammatory drug (NSAID) as this increases the risk of side effects. Aspirin may decrease the amount of fenbufen in the blood if taken at the same time. Fenbufen should not be taken with quinolone antibiotics such as enoxacin, ofloxacin or ciprofloxacin, as it may increase the potential for side effects such as convulsions.

Fenbufen may decrease the removal of methotrexate from the body, resulting in an increased risk of methotrexate related side effects.

If fenbufen is taken with warfarin there may be an increased risk of side effects such as stomach or intestinal bleeding. Fenbufen may also cause a minor increase in bleeding time (prothrombin time), but this is unlikely to be significant. However people stabilised on anticoagulants such as warfarin should have their prothrombin time monitored if fenbufen is added to treatment.

Other NSAIDs have been reported to cause an increase in the amount of lithium in the blood. This has not been reported with fenbufen, but people who are stabilised on lithium should have their lithium levels monitored if fenbufen is added to treatment.

The manufacturer of mifeprostone recommends that NSAIDs such as fenbufen should not be used within 8-12 days of taking mifeprostone.

There may be an increased risk of kidney problems if fenbufen is taken with cyclosporin, diuretics or ACE inhibitors. There may be an increased risk of stomach or intestinal side effects if fenbufen is taken with corticosteroids such as prednisolone.

Adverse Drug Reaction

Current or previous peptic ulcer

People in whom aspirin or other medicines in this class (NSAIDs), cause attacks of asthma, itchy rash (urticaria) or nasal inflammation (rhinitis).

Suspected peptic ulcer

This medicine should not be used if you are allergic to one or any of its ingredients. Please inform doctor or pharmacist if person have previously experienced such an allergy.

Pregnancy and Breastfeeding : certain medicines should not be used during pregnancy or breastfeeding. However, other medicines may be safely used in pregnancy or breastfeeding providing the benefits to the mother outweigh the risks to the unborn baby.

Side Effects

Medicines and their possible side effects can affect individual people in different ways. The following are some of the side effects that are known to be associated with this medicine.

Rash, Disturbed sleep, Blood disorders, Disturbances of the gut such as diarrhoea, constipation, nausea, vomiting or abdominal pain, Lung disorders, Visual disturbances, Indigestion (dyspepsia), Abnormal reaction of the skin to light, usually a rash (photosensitivity), Retention of water in the body tissues (fluid retention), resulting in swelling (oedema), Dizziness, Kidney damage, Severe blistering skin reaction affecting the tissues of the eyes, mouth, throat and genitals.(Stevens-Johnson Syndrome), Liver disorders, Hypersensitivity reactions such as narrowing of the airways (bronchospasm), swelling of the lips, throat and tongue (angioedema) or severe skin reaction (toxic epidermal necrolysis), Ulceration or bleeding of the stomach or intestines.

Dosage

Orally for adults 300 mg per day, 3 times a day during meals. In long-term treatment 2 times a day 300 mg, or once 600 mg in the evening. It is advised not to exceed daily dosage over 900 mg.

Theraputic Uses

A form of arthritis (ankylosing spondylitis) inflammatory disease of the joints Musculoskeletal disorders such as tendon inflammation (tendinitis), sprains, strains, dislocations and fractures.

Brand Name

USA - Tab. Lederfen

INDIA - Tab. Lederfen

Flurbiprofen

Description

Flurbiprofen is a member of the phenylalkanoic acid derivative group of nonsteroidal anti-inflammatory drugs. Flurbiprofen is a racemic mixture of (+)S- and (−)R-enantiomers. Flurbiprofen is a white or slightly yellow crystalline powder. It is slightly soluble in water at pH 7.0 and readily soluble in most polar solvents.

Molecular weight - 244.27

Melting point – 114 ~ 117°C

Solubility : Freely soluble in Ethanol (95%), in chloroform and in Ether practically insoluble in water

Half life : Plasma half life, 2 ~ 6h (mean 3.5)

Pharmacodynamics

Flurbiprofen is a nonsteroidal anti-inflammatory drug that exhibits anti-inflammatory, analgesic, and antipyretic activities in animal models. The mechanism of action of NSAID, like that of other nonsteroidal anti-inflammatory drugs, is not completely understood but may be related to prostaglandin synthetase inhibition.

Pharmacokinetics

Absorption

The mean oral bioavailability of flurbiprofen Tablet 100 mg is 96% relative to an oral solution. Flurbiprofen is rapidly and non-stereoselectively absorbed from NSAID, with peak plasma concentrations occurring at about 2 hours. Administration of NSAID with either food or antacids may alter the rate but not the extent of flurbiprofen absorption.

Distribution

The apparent volume of distribution of both R- and S-flurbiprofen is approximately 0.12 L/Kg. Both flurbiprofen enantiomers are more than 99% bound to plasma proteins, primarily albumin. Plasma protein binding is relatively constant for the typical average steady-state concentrations (≤10 µg/mL) achieved with recommended doses. Flurbiprofen is poorly excreted into human milk. The nursing infant dose is predicted to be approximately 0.1 mg/day in the established milk of a woman taking NSAID 200 mg/day.

Metabolism

Several flurbiprofen metabolites have been identified in human plasma and urine. These metabolites include 4'-hydroxy-flurbiprofen, 3', 4'-dihydroxy-flurbiprofen, 3'-hydroxy-4'-methoxyflurbiprofen, their conjugates, and conjugated flurbiprofen. Unlike other arylpropionic acid derivatives (eg, ibuprofen), metabolism of R-flurbiprofen to S-flurbiprofen is minimal. In vitro studies have demonstrated that cytochrome P450 2C9 plays an important role in the metabolism of flurbiprofen to its major metabolite, 4'-hydroxy-flurbiprofen. The 4'-hydroxy-flurbiprofen metabolite showed little anti-inflammatory activity in animal models of inflammation. Flurbiprofen does not induce enzymes that alter its metabolism.

The total plasma clearance of unbound flurbiprofen is not stereoselective, and clearance of flurbiprofen is independent of dose when used within the therapeutic range.

Excretion

Less than 3% of flurbiprofen is excreted unchanged in the urine, with about 70% of the dose eliminated in the urine as parent drug and metabolites. Because renal elimination is a significant pathway of elimination of flurbiprofen metabolites, dosing adjustment in patients with moderate or severe renal dysfunction may be necessary to avoid accumulation of flurbiprofen metabolites. The mean terminal disposition half-lives ($t\frac{1}{2}$) of R- and S-flurbiprofen are similar, about 4.7 and 5.7 hours, respectively. There is little accumulation of flurbiprofen following multiple doses of NSAID.

Drug Interactions

Cimetidine, Ranitidine: In normal volunteers, pretreatment with cimetidine or ranitidine did not affect flurbiprofen pharmacokinetics, except for a small (13%) but statistically significant increase in the area under the serum concentration curve of flurbiprofen in subjects who received cimetidine.

Digoxin : Concomitant administration of flurbiprofen and digoxin did not change the steady state serum levels of either drug.

Diuretics : Studies in healthy volunteers have shown that, like other nonsteroidal anti-inflammatory drugs, flurbiprofen can interfere with the effects of furosemide. Although results have varied from study to study, effects have been shown on furosemide-stimulated diuresis, natriuresis, and kaliuresis.

Lithium : NSAIDs have produced an elevation of plasma lithium levels and a reduction in renal lithium clearance. The mean minimum lithium concentration increased 15% and the renal clearance was decreased by approximately 20%. These effects have been attributed to inhibition of renal prostaglandin synthesis by the nonsteroidal anti-inflammatory drug. Thus, when nonsteroidal anti-inflammatory drugs and lithium are administered concurrently, subjects should be observed carefully for signs of lithium toxicity.

Methotrexate : Coadministration of methotrexate (10 to 25 mg/dose) and NSAID (300 mg/day) resulted in no observable interaction between these two drugs.

ACE-inhibitors : Nonsteroidal anti-inflammatory drugs may diminish the antihypertensive effect of ACE-inhibitors. This interaction should be given consideration in patients taking nonsteroidal anti-inflammatory drugs concomitantly with ACE-inhibitors.

Anticoagulants : The effects of warfarin and NSAIDs on GI bleeding are synergistic, such that users of both drugs together have a risk of serious GI bleeding higher than users of either drug alone. The physician should be cautious when administering NSAID to patients taking warfarin or other anticoagulants.

Aspirin : Concurrent administration of aspirin lowers serum flurbiprofen concentrations. The clinical significance of this interaction is not known; however, as with other NSAIDs, concomitant administration of flurbiprofen and aspirin is not generally recommended because of the potential for increased adverse effects.

Beta-adrenergic blocking agents : Flurbiprofen attenuated the hypotensive effect of propranolol but not atenolol. The mechanism underlying this interference is unknown. Patients taking both flurbiprofen and a beta-blocker should be monitored to ensure that a satisfactory hypotensive effect is achieved.

Diuretics : NSAIDs can reduce the natriuretic effect-of furosemide and thiazides in some patients. This response has been attributed to inhibition of renal prostaglandin synthesis. During concomitant therapy with NSAIDs, the patient should be observed closely for signs of renal failure as well as diuretic efficacy.

Side Effect

Serious side effects include heart attack, stroke, high blood pressure, heart failure from body swelling (fluid retention), kidney problems including kidney failure, bleeding and ulcers in the stomach and intestine, low red blood cells (anemia), life-threatening skin reactions, life-threatening allergic reactions, liver problems including liver failure, asthma attacks in people who have asthma.

Other side effects include

Stomach pain, constipation, diarrhea, gas, heartburn, nausea, vomiting, dizziness.

Skin Reactions

NSAIDs can cause serious skin adverse events such as exfoliative dermatitis, Steven-Johnson Syndrom (SJS), and toxic epidermal necrolysis (TEN), which can be fatal. These serious events may occur without warning. Patients should be informed about the signs and symptoms of serious skin manifestations and use of the drug should be discontinued at the first appearance of skin rash or any other sign of hypersensitivity.

Pregnancy

In late pregnancy, as with other NSAIDs, NSAID should be avoided because it may cause premature closure of the ductus arteriosus.

Adverse Reactions

Teratogenic effects: Pregnancy Category C

Reproductive studies conducted in rats and rabbits have not demonstrated evidence of developmental abnormalities. However, animal reproduction studies are not always predictive of human response. There are no adequate and well-controlled studies in pregnant women. NSAID should be used in pregnancy only if the potential benefit justifies the potential risk to the fetus.

Nonteratogenic effects

Because of the known effects of nonsteroidal anti-inflammatory drugs on the fetal cardiovascular system (closure of ductus arteriosus), use during late pregnancy should be avoided.

Labor and Delivery

In rat studies with nonsteroidal anti-inflammatory drugs, as with other drugs known to inhibit prostaglandin synthesis, an increased incidence of dystocia, delayed parturition, and decreased pup survival occurred. The effects of NSAID on labor and delivery in pregnant women are unknown.

Nursing Mothers

Concentrations of flurbiprofen in breast milk and plasma of nursing mothers suggest that a nursing infant could receive approximately 0.10 mg flurbiprofen per day in the established milk of a woman taking NSAID 200 mg/day. Because of possible adverse effects of prostaglandin-inhibiting drugs on neonates, a decision should be made whether to discontinue nursing or to discontinue the drug, taking into account the importance of the drug to the mother.

Pediatric Use

Safety and effectiveness in pediatric patients have not been established.

Dosage and Administration

150-200mg Daily to 300mg Daily

Carefully consider the potential benefits and risks of NSAID and other treatment options before deciding to use NSAID. Use the lowest effective dose for the shortest duration consistent with individual patient treatment goals.

After observing the response to initial therapy with NSAID, the dose and frequency should be adjusted to suit an individual patient's needs. For relief of the signs and symptoms of rheumatoid arthritis or osteoarthritis, the recommended starting dose of NSAID is 200 to 300 mg per day, divided for administration two, three, or four times a day. The largest recommended single dose in a multiple-dose daily regimen is 100 mg.

Therapeutic Uses

A form of arthritis (ankylosing spondylitis) inflammatory disease of the joints Musculoskeletal disorders such as tendon inflammation (tendinitis), sprains, strains, dislocations and fractures

Brand Name

> **India** Flur IVA remedies EYE drop, FBN DPS microvision, OCUFLUR FDC

> **USA** Tab. Ocufen

Ketoprofen

Description

White to off white, odorless, crystalline, and non-hygroscopic, melts about 95^0C. It is practically insoluble in water, soluble in fixed bases, freely soluble in alcohol, chloroform, acetone, ether.

Chemistry

Ketoprofen is a racemic mixture; in animal studies the S-(+) enantiomer, dextro ketoprofen has approximately twice the analgesic activity of ketoprofen by weigh. Placing the phenoxy group in the ortho- or para-position of the arylpropionic ring markedly decreases activity. Replacement of the carbonyl group with an oxygen bridge between two aromatic rings yields an analogue (fenoprofen) which also marketed.

Chemical structure

Molecular formula - $C_{16}H_{14}O_3$

Pharmacodynemics

Ketoprofen have three major pharmacologically desirable actions, all of which results from the inhibition of arachidonic acid cyclooxygenase in inflammatory cells (the COX2 isoenzyme), and the resultant decrease in prostanoid synthesis.

Ketoprofen inhibits the synthesis of leukotrienes and leukocyte migration into inflamed joints in addition to inhibiting the biosynthesis of prostaglandins. It stabilizes the lysosomal membrane during inflammation resulting in decreased tissue destruction. Antibradykinin activity has also been observed. Bradykinin is released during inflammation and can activate peripheral pain receptors. In addition to anti-inflammatory activity, ketoprofen also possesses antipyretic and analgesic activity. Although it is less potent than indomethacin as an anti-inflammatory agent and as an analgesic, its ability to produce gastric lesions is about the same.

Pharmacokinetics

Absorption

Ketoprofen is rapidly absorbed after oral administration. Food reduces the rate of absorption but not extent of absorption.

Distribution

Maximal concentration in plasma is achieved within 1 to 2 hours .The drug is extensively bound to plasma proteins (90%).

Metabolism

Ketoprofen has a half-life in plasma of about 2 hours. Slightly longer half-lives are observed in elderly subjects. Ketoprofen is conjugated with glucuronic acid in the liver. As steady state, which may take several day to achieve the accumulation half life is about 25hour 600mg daily and 21hour after 1200mg daily.

Metabolism of ketoprofen is due to two major processes, a hydroxylation process predominant to the rat, although the preferred excretory from in the rat is unchanged ketoprofen and glucuronide conjugation in other species including man .The glucuronide conjugation is predominant in the rabbit and man but in the hydroxylation is not totally absent.

Excretion

Ketoprofen is excreted in the urine. Patients with impaired renal function eliminate the drug more slowly. The kinetics of elimination is 1st order and the rate constant is 0.350 hours.

Dosage and Administration

Ketoprofen is available as capsules and tablets (25mg & 50mg), with a recommended daily dose of 150mg to 300mg divided into three or four doses. It is also available as extended –release capsules (100mg, 150mg and 200mg).

Toxic Effects

Dyspepsia and other gastrointestinal side effects have been observed in about 30% of patients, but these side effects are generally mild and are less frequent than those in patients treated with aspirin. Untoward effects are reduced when the drug is taken with food, milk, or antacids. Ketoprofen can cause fluid retention and increased plasma concentration of creatinine. These effects are generally transient and occur in the absence of symptoms, but they are more common in patients who are receiving diuretics or in those over the age of 60.Renal function should be monitored in such patients.

When ketoprofen is administered intramuscularly there may be at injection site and occasionally tissue damage. Ketoprofen suppositories may cause local irritation. Ketoprofen, Dex ketoprofen should be used with caution in patients with renal hepatic impairment.

In some countries ketoprofen is considered to be contraindicated in patients with heart failure. However evidence that keroprofen is any more likely than other NSAIDs to precipitate or to aggravate heart failure seems to be lacking.

Hypersensitivity : Life threatening asthma, urticaria, and angioedema developed. Cardic and respiratory arrest occurred in an asthmatic patient shortly after taking ketoprofen.

Myasthenia gravis : There has been an brief report of a single dose of ketoprofen 50mg by mouth precipitating a cholinergic crisis in a patient with well controlled myasthenia gravis.

Other main adverse effects are pancreatitis, photosensitivity, and renal impairment.

Drug and Food Interaction of Ketoprofen

Probenacid : delays the excretion of ketoprofen and decrease its extent of protein binding resulting in increase plasma ketoprofen concentration.

Metolazone : Reduced urinary potassium and chloride excretion.

Aspirin : Decreased protein-binding and increased plasma clearance of ketoprofen

Bendroflumethiazide : Reduced urinary potassium and chloride excretion.

Bumetanide : Potassium and chloride Reduced urinary excretion.

Chlorothiazide : Reduced urinary potassium and chloride excretion.

Chlorthalidone : Reduced urinary potassium and chloride excretion.

Ethacrynic Acid : Reduced urinary potassium and chloride excretion.

Furosemide : Reduced urinary potassium and chloride excretion.

Hydrochlorothiazide : Reduced urinary potassium and chloride excretion.

Hydroflumethiazide : Reduced urinary potassium and chloride excretion.

Indapamide : Reduced urinary potassium and chloride excretion.

Lithium Carbonate : Increased steady-state plasma lithium levels.

Lithium Citrate : Increased steady-state plasma lithium levels.

Amiloride Hydrochloride : Reduced urinary potassium and chloride excretion.

Warfarin Sodium : Concurrent therapy requires close monitoring of patients on both drugs.

Methotrexate Sodium : Increased toxicity; avoid coadministration.

Polythiazide : Reduced urinary potassium and chloride excretion.

Uses and Administration

- Ketoprofen is used in musculoskeletal and joint disorder such as ankylosing spondylitis, osteoarthritis, and rheumatoid arthritis.

- It is also used in peri articular disorder such as bursitis and tendonitis.

- It is used in dysmenorrhoea, postoperative pain and painful and inflammatory condition such as acute gout or soft tissue disorder.

- Ketoprofen may be given by deep intramascular injection into the glutted muscle for acute exacerbation of masculoskeletal, joint peri-articular and soft tissue disorder.

Marketed Preparation

USA - Actron, Orudis, Oruvail

Canada - Apoketo, Novoketo

Hongkong - Fastum, Orudis Oruvail

Italy - Alket, Desketo

Israel - Ketonail, Profenid

N Z - Kefen

Australia - Orudis, Oruvail

Austria - Actron, Keprodol

U K – Fenoket, Iomethid

Oxaprozin

History

Oxaprozin is a nonsteroidal anti-inflammatory drug characterised by a propionic acid-based structure. It is able to diffuse easily into inflamed synovial tissues after oral administration. Although discovered more than 20 years ago, it is now under intensive investigation because of its unusual pharmacodynamic properties. Other than being a nonselective cyclooxygenase inhibitor.

Description

Oxaprozin is a nonsteroidal anti-inflammatory drug (NSAID), chemically designated as 4,5-diphenyl-2-oxazole-propionic acid, and has the following chemical structure: The empirical formula for oxaprozin is $C_{18}H_{15}NO_3$, and the molecular weight is 293. Oxaprozin is a white to off-white powder with a slight odor and a melting point of 162^0C to 163^0C. It is slightly soluble in alcohol and insoluble in water, with an octanol/water partition coefficient of 4.8 at physiologic pH (7.4). The pK_a in water is 4.3.

IUPAC name - 4,5-Diphenyl-2Oxazolepropionic acid.

Chemical Formula - $C_{15}H_{18}N\,O_3$

Chemical Structure

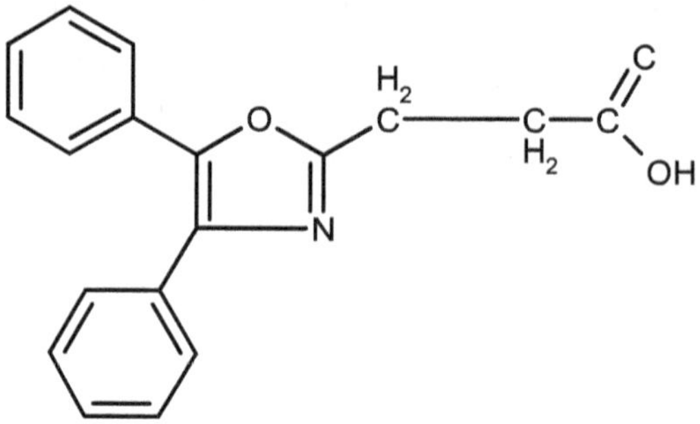

Pharmacodynamic

Oxaprozin is a nonselective cyclooxygenase inhibitor, the drug is capable of inhibiting both anandamide hydrolase in neurons (median inhibitory concentration [IC50] = 85 micromol/l), with consequent potent analgesic activity, and NF-kappaB activation in inflammatory cells (IC50 = 50 micromol/l). Moreover, oxaprozin induces apoptosis of activated monocytes in a dose-dependent manner, with the effect being detectable at a concentration of 5 micromol/l and reaching the maximum activity at 50 micromol/l. As monocyte-macrophages and NF-kappaB pathways are crucial for synthesis of proinflammatory and histotoxic mediators in inflamed joints, oxaprozin appears to be endowed with pharmacodynamic properties exceeding those presently assumed as markers of classical nonsteroidal anti-inflammatory drug.

Machanism of Action

Oxaprozin eye drops significantly reduced the signs of ocular inflammation elicited by sodium arachidonate on conjunctiva and iris. Oxaprozin treatment significantly reduced the levels of polymorphonuclear leukocytes and protein concentration in aqueous samples obtained from the eyes treated with arachidonate. Present data suggest, for the first time, that oxaprozin may be employed topically to prevent ocular reactions where the arachidonic acid cascade is activated.

Pharmacokinetics

Absorption

Oxaprozin is well absorbed orally. It is slowly but extensively absorbed from gastrointestinal tract. Oxaprozin is 95% absorbed after oral administration. Food may reduce the rate of absorption of Oxaprozin, but the extent of absorption is unchanged. Antacids do not significantly affect the extent and rate of Oxaprozin absorption.

Distribution

Oxaprozin is highly bound to plasma protein and peak plasma concentration achieved in 3 to 6 hours. The apparent volume of distribution (Vd/F) of total Oxaprozin is approximately 11–17 L/70 kg. Oxaprozin is 99% bound to plasma proteins, primarily to albumin. At therapeutic drug concentrations, the plasma protein binding of Oxaprozin is saturable, resulting in a higher proportion of the free drug as the total drug concentration is increased.

Metabolism

Oxaprozin is highly bound to plasma protein and peak plasma concentration achieved in 3 to 6 hours. The drug is metabolized in the liver by microsomal oxidation and conjugation with glucuronic acid to form inactive metabolites, which are excreted in the urine and faeces.

Excretion

It primarily eliminated by urinary excretion. The half-life is 40 to60 hours, & this increases with age. Approximately 5% of the Oxaprozin dose is excreted unchanged in the urine. Sixty-five percent (65%) of the dose is excreted in the urine and 35% in the feces as metabolite. Biliary excretion of unchanged Oxaprozin is a minor pathway, and enterohepatic recycling of Oxaprozin is insignificant.

Drug Interaction

Food, unspecified : Reduces the rate of absorption of oxaprozin, but the extent of absorption is unchanged.

Warfarin Sodium : Co-administration with 1200 mg/day of Daypro does not affect anticoagulant effects of warfarin; however, caution should be exercised.

Ranitidine Hydrochloride : Concurrent use may reduce the total body clearance of oxaprozin.

Cimetidine Hydrochloride : Concurrent use may reduce the total body clearance of oxaprozin.

Cimetidine : Concurrent use may reduce the total body clearance of oxaprozin).

Aspirin : Co-administration is not recommended because oxaprozin displaces salicylates from binding sites resulting in increased risk of salicylate toxicity).

Adverse Drug Reaction

Gastrointestinal Disturbances – This result mainly from inhibition of COX-1. COX-1 action is responsible for the synthesis of the prostaglandins that normally inhibit acid secretion, as well as having a protective action on the mucosa. Common GIT side effects are dyspepsia, diarrhea, nausea, and vomiting and in somecases, gastric bleeding and ulceration. Skin Reactions the type of skin condition seen varies from mild rashes, urticaria and photosensitivity reaction.

Adverse Renal Effects Therapeutic dose of oxaprozin in hralthy individuals pose little threat to kidney function, but in susceptible patients they cause acute renal insufficicncy, which is reversible stooping the drug.

Other Unwanted Effects Unwanted effects of oxaprozin include bone marrow disturbances and liver disorders m the latter more likely if there is already renal impairment.

Dosage and Administration

1200mg daily once by mouth in the form of tablet in severe osteoarthritis and rheumatoid arthritis. 600mg daily in mild osteoarthritis and rheumatoid arthritis. In osteoarthritis and rheumatoid arthritis and juvenile rheumatoid arthritis, the dosage should be individualized to the lowest effective dose of Oxaprozin to minimize adverse effects.

Cinical Efficacy

Both oxaprozin and diclofenac compared well in the primary study endpoint of reduction in shoulder pain. Oxaprozin and diclofenac were well tolerated and oxaprozin showed better improvement in shoulder function and in the mental health item of the SF-36 quality of life component. The study by Heller and Tarricone is an addition to the large number of clinical trials which demonstrate that oxaprozin has equal efficacy in comparison with standard doses of commonly used anti-rheumatic agents such as aspirin, diclofenac, ibuprofen, indomethacin etc. in several different painful musculoskeletal conditions.

Therapeutic Uses

- Oxaprozin's strong analgesic qualities are particularly useful in painful musculoskeletal conditions such as periarthritis of the shoulder

- Oxaprozin is effective in models of inflammation, pain and pyrexia
- Oxaprozin is effective and well tolerated in the clinical management of adult rheumatoid arthritis (RA), osteoarthritis (OA), ankylosing spondylitis, soft tissue disorders and postoperative dental pain

Brand Names-

Canada - Daypro

U S A - Daypro

South Africa – DEFLAM.

Fenoprofen

Description

Fenoprofen is a nonsteroidal anti-inflammatory drug (NSAID) of the propionic acid chemical class. Fenoprofen possesses antipyretic and analgesic properties and is structurally and pharmacologically related to ibuprofen and naproxen. All NSAIDs including fenoprofen cause an increased risk of serious gastrointestinal adverse effects including bleeding, ulceration, and perforation of the stomach or intestines and may cause an increased risk of serious cardiovascular thrombotic events, myocardial infarction, and stroke. The lowest effective fenoprofen dose for the shortest possible duration is recommended, as the risk for adverse effects may increase with duration of use. Fenoprofen is indicated for the symptomatic treatment of rheumatoid arthritis and osteoarthritis, and to alleviate mild to moderate pain. Clinical trials have demonstrated some effectiveness in acute gouty arthritis and ankylosing spondylitis.

Chemical Structure

Chemistry

Fenoprofen has an asymmetric centre which allows the existence of two enantiomers (R) (-) and (S) (+). Recently the resolved R and S isomers and RS racemates of fenoprofen were compared in vitro as inhibitors of fatty acids cyclooxygenase system from human platelets which is often used to detect drugs that have an anti inflammatory activity associated with inhibition of prostaglandin synthesis. On the basis of 0% inhibition one isomer was found to be 2 times more active than racemates and 35 times more active than other isomer.

Several fenoprofen salts were prepared to obtain the most acceptable form for an oral dosage formulation. Thermal analysis techniques were used to compare stabilities of the water of hydration in different salt forms and to assess the effects of the water of hydration on compatibility with propoxyphene and codeine salts. Photodegradation products of fenoprofen were isolated and identified, and their relevance to product form.

Pharmacodynamics

Fenoprofen inhibits prostaglandin synthesis by decreasing the activity of the enzyme cyclooxygenase which results is decreased formation of prostaglandin precursors. Fenoprofen competitively inhibits both cyclooxygcnasc (COX) isoenzymes, COX-1 and COX-2, by blocking arachidonate binding resulting in analgesic, antipyretic, and anti-inflammatory pharmacologic effects. The enzymes COX-1 and COX-2 catalyze the conversion of arachidonic acid to prostaglandin G_2 (PGG_2), the first step of the synthesis prostaglandins and thromboxanes that are involved in rapid physiological responses. COX isoenzymes are also responsible for a peroxidase reaction, which is not affected by NSAIDs. In addition, NSAIDs do not suppress leukotriene synthesis by lipoxygenase pathways. COX-1 is constitutively expressed in almost all tissues, while COX-2 appears to only be constitutively expressed in the brain, kidney, bones, reproductive organs, and some neoplasms (e.g., colon and prostate cancers). COX-1 is responsible for prostaglandin synthesis in response to stimulation by circulating hormones, as well as maintenance of normal renal function, gastric mucosal integrity, and hemostasis. However, COX-2 is inducible in many cells in response to certain mediators of inflammation (e.g., interleukin-1, tumor necrosis factor, lipopolysaccharide, mitogens, and reactive oxygen intermediates).

Pharmacokinetics

Fenoprofen is rapidly and almost completely absorbed from the GI tract. When fenoprofen is taken with food, the peak plasma concentration is delayed and decreased. Peak plasma concentrations are achieved about 2 hours after oral administration. The onset of analgesic activity occurs within 15-30 minutes, and the duration of action is 4-6 hours. Fenoprofen is approximately 99% protein-bound. It does not appear to cross the placenta, and concentrations in breast milk are less than 2% of maternal plasma concentrations. The plasma half-life is 2.5-3 hours. Fenoprofen is hepatically metabolized to 4-hydroxyfenoprofen, which is thought to be inactive. Glucuronic acid conjugates of the drug and metabolite are also formed. Fenoprofen appears to undergo enterohepatic circulation. Elimination occurs predominantly through renal excretion, with 90% of a dose appearing as glucuronides and other conjugates. Only 2—5% is excreted as unchanged fenoprofen. A small amount of the drug is excreted in the feces. Dosage adjustments for renal impairment are not available, but do not appear to be necessary.

Absorption : Rapidly absorbed under fasting conditions, and peak plasma levels of 50 µg/mL are achieved within 2 hours after oral administration of 600 mg doses.

Protein binding : - 99% to albumin

Clinical Efficacy

Fenoprofen (dl-2-[3-phenoxyphenyl]propionic acid) is a new non-steroidal anti-inflammatory, antipyretic, analgesic agent advocated for use in rheumatoid arthritis, degenerative joint disease, ankylosing spondylitis and gout. Published data suggest that in rheumatoid arthritis, fenoprofen 2.4 g daily is comparable in effectiveness with moderate doses of aspirin (3.6 to 4 g daily), but generally causes fewer and milder side-effects at the dosages used. In published comparisons with other non-steroidal anti-inflammatory agents of the same chemical group, it is closely comparable with naproxen in effectiveness but tends to cause more minor side-effects than naproxen. However, as no one of the non-steroidal anti-inflammatory agents is the most suitable drug for all patients requiring such therapy, fenoprofen should be considered along with the other drugs of its type in the initial treatment of the arthritic patient. Fenoprofen has compared favorably with phenylbutazone in osteoarthrosis of the hips and with aspirin in osteoarthrosis of the shoulders, hips, knees and spine.

Side effects

Fenoprofen may cause side effects. The most frequently reported side effects have been gastrointestinal ones. Abdominal discomfort and dyspepsia occurs in about 15% patiens. These side effects are almost less intense than with equieffective doses of aspirin and force of discontinuation of therapy in a small percentage of patients.other side effects include:-

- headache
- nervousness
- drowsiness
- sweating

- constipation
- ringing in the ear

Adverse Reaction

Central nervous system : Dizziness (7% to 15%), somnolence (9% to 15%)

Gastrointestinal : Abdominal cramps (2% to 4%), heartburn, indigestion, nausea (8% to 14%), dyspepsia (10% to 14%), flatulence (14%), anorexia (14%), constipation (7% to 14%), occult blood in stool (14%), vomiting (3% to 14%), diarrhea (2% to 14%).

Dermatologic : Itching

Endocrine & metabolic : Fluid retention

Drug Interactions

- *ACE inhibitors :* Antihypertensive effects may be decreased by concurrent therapy with NSAIDs; monitor blood pressure.

- *Angiotensin II antagonists :* Antihypertensive effects may be decreased by concurrent therapy with NSAIDs; monitor blood pressure.

- Anticoagulants (warfarin, heparin, LMWHs) in combination with NSAIDs can cause increased risk of bleeding.

- Other antiplatelet drugs (ticlopidine, clopidogrel, aspirin, abciximab, dipyridamole, eptifibatide, tirofiban) can cause an increased risk of bleeding.

- Cholestyramine and colestipol reduce the bioavailability of diclofenac; separate administration times.

- Corticosteroids may increase the risk of GI ulceration; avoid concurrent use.

- *Cyclosporine :* NSAIDs may increase serum creatinine, potassium, blood pressure, and cyclosporine levels; monitor cyclosporine levels and renal function carefully.

- Gentamicin and amikacin serum concentrations are increased by indomethacin in premature infants. Results may apply to other aminoglycosides and NSAIDs.

- Hydralazine's antihypertensive effect is decreased; avoid concurrent use.

- Lithium levels can be increased; avoid concurrent use if possible or monitor lithium levels and adjust dose. Sulindac may have the least effect. When NSAID is stopped, lithium will need adjustment again.

- Loop diuretics efficacy (diuretic and antihypertensive effect) is reduced. Indomethacin reduces this efficacy; however, it may be anticipated with any NSAID.
- *Methotrexate* : Severe bone marrow suppression, aplastic anemia, and GI toxicity have been reported with concomitant NSAID therapy. Avoid use during moderate or high-dose methotrexate (increased and prolonged methotrexate levels). NSAID use during low-dose treatment of rheumatoid arthritis has not been fully evaluated; extreme caution is warranted.
- Verapamil plasma concentration is decreased by diclofenac; avoid concurrent use.
- Warfarin's INRs may be increased by piroxicam. Other NSAIDs may have the same effect depending on dose and duration. Monitor INR closely. Use the lowest dose of NSAIDs possible and for the briefest duration.

Indoprofen

Description

Indoprofen (INP) is a nonsteroidal anti-inflammatory drug which was used in the treatment of both osteoarthritis and rheumatoid arthritis. It is a new propionic acid derivative [4(1-oxo-2-iso indolinyl) phenyl propionic acid]. It has potent analgesic, anti inflammatory and antipyretic activity. Despite the structural analogy, few in vitro investigations about photophysical and photochemical properties of INP have been published. It has been reported that contrary to most NSAID this compound does not induce inflammatory reaction under irradiation. However, peroxide formation during irradiation under oxygen and lipid photoperoxidation has been shown to occur. Nevertheless, no data exists in the literature concerning its photochemistry in aqueous or organic solutions. Thus, the purpose of the present study is on the one hand to establish the excited-state properties of INP and, on the other hand, to investigate its photoreactivity in different media, both under aerobic and anaerobic conditions.

Structure of Indoprofen

Mechanism of Action

Indoprofen upregulates the survival motor neuron protein through a cyclooxygenase independent mechanism. Spinal muscular atrophy (SMA) is an auto somal recessive disease characterized by rapid degeneration of lower motor neuron in the anterior horn of the spinal cord due to reduced survival motor neuron protein. Indoprofen selectively upregulated this SMN reporter activity.

Pharmacokinetics

Indoprofen is well absorbed from the stomach, highly protein bound and excreted mainly in the urine as the glucuronides. Peak plasma levels are reached with in 30 mins of an oral dose of 100 mg and the compound has a short plasma half life of about 3hrs in patient. The pharmacokinetics of indoprofen was investigated in several studies in healthy volunteers and in rheumatoid arthritis patients. In healthy subjects the drug is rapidly eliminated with a biological half-life of 2.3 h. The drug and its metabolites are almost completely excreted in urine within 24 h from administration. The absorption of indoprofen administered orally to fasting subjects as 100 mg capsules and 200 mg tablets is rapid and complete. The bioavailability of indoprofen tablets is not adversely affected by the presence of food in the gastrointestinal tract. Following administration of 600 mg of indoprofen per day for 7 days, no changes are observed in the drug plasma level profile. There are no substantial differences between healthy subjects and rheumatoid arthritis patients as regards the pharmacokinetics properties of oral indoprofen.

Side Effects

As an anti-inflammatory, indoprofen (200 mg four times daily) was superior to both ibuprofen (300 mg four times daily) and placebo. With regular administration, the effect of indoprofen reached a plateau within 24 hours of the start of treatment. Long term administration confirmed the safety of indoprofen and the overall incidence of side effects was similar to that associated with ibuprofen therapy.

Naproxen

Description

Naproxen is a proprionic acid derivative related to the arylacetic acid group of nonsteroidal anti-inflammatory drugs. The chemical names for naproxen and naproxen sodium are (S)-6-methoxy-O-methyl-2-naphthaleneacetic acid and (S)-6-methoxy O-methyl-2-naphthaleneacetic acid, sodium salt, respectively.

Molecular weight - 230.26

Molecular formula - $C_{14}H_{14}O_3$

Naproxen is an odorless, white to off-white crystalline substance. It is lipid-soluble, practically insoluble in water at low pH and freely soluble in water at high pH. The octanol/water partition coefficient of naproxen at pH 7.4 is 1.6 to 1.8. Naproxen sodium is a white to creamy white, crystalline solid, freely soluble in water at neutral pH.

Pharmacodynamics

Naproxen is a nonsteroidal anti-inflammatory (NSAID) with analgesic, anti-inflammatory and antipyretic properties. The onset of pain relief is more rapid with naproxen sodium than with naproxen, therefore naproxen sodium is recommended for the management of acute painful conditions.Naproxen is a propionic acid derivative related to the arylacetic acid class of medicines. The chemical name of naproxen is (+)-6-methoxy-alpha-methyl-2-naphthaleneacetic acid. It is an odourless, white to off-white crystalline substance. It is lipid soluble, practically insoluble in water at low pH and freely soluble in water at high pH. Naproxen sodium is a white to creamy white, crystalline solid, freely soluble in water at neutral pH.

Naproxen belongs to a class of drugs called non–steroidal anti-inflamaory drus. Naproxen works by reducing the levels of prostaglanding, chemicals that are responsible for pain, fever, inflammation. Naproxen blocks the enzyme that makes prostaglandins [cyclooxygenase], resulting in lower concentrations of prostaglandins. As a consequence, inflammation, pain and fever are reduced. Naproxen was approved by the FDA in December

1991.Naproxen has been shown to have striking anti-inflammatory properties when tested in human clinical studies and classical animal test systems. In addition, it has marked analgesic and antipyretic actions. It exhibits its anti-inflammatory effects even in adrenalectomised animals, indicating that its action is not mediated through the pituitary axis. It inhibits synthesis of prostaglandins. As with other similar agents, however, the exact mechanism of its anti-inflammatory action is not known.

Pharmacokinetics

Absorption : Naproxen and naproxen sodium are rapidly and completely absorbed from the gastrointestinal tract after oral administration. Naproxen sodium is more rapidly absorbed than naproxen. Concomitant administration of food can delay the absorption of naproxen and naproxen sodium, but does not affect its extent.

Distribution : Naproxen has a volume of distribution of 0.16 l/kg. At therapeutic levels naproxen is greater than 99% albumin-bound. At doses of naproxen greater than 500 mg/day, there is less than proportional increase in plasma levels due to an increase in clearance caused by saturation of plasma protein binding at higher doses. However, the concentration of unbound naproxen continues to increase proportionally to dose.

Steady state plasma level of naproxen are reached after 3-4 days. Naproxen enters synovial fluid, crosses the placenta and has been found in the milk of lactating mothers at a concentration approximately 1% of that found in plasma.

Metabolism : Naproxen is extensively metabolised in the liver to 6-0-desmethyl naproxen.

Elimination : Approximately 95% of the naproxen from any dose is excreted in the urine, primarily as naproxen (less than 1%), 6-0-desmethyl naproxen (less than 1%), or their conjugates (66 - 92%). The rate of excretion of metabolites and conjugates has been found to coincide closely with the rate of naproxen disappearance from the plasma. Small amounts, 3% or less, are excreted in the faeces.

The clearance of naproxen is approximately 0.13 mL/min/kg. The elimination half-life of naproxen is approximately 14 hours and is independent of the chemical form or the formulation.

Side Effects

Blood in vomit or bloody, black, or tarry stools. These symptoms could indicate damage to the stomach or intestines, which could be dangerous. An allergic reaction (difficulty breathing; closing of the throat; swelling of the lips, tongue, or face; or hives); muscle cramps, numbness, or tingling; ulcers (open sores) in the mouth; rapid weight gain (fluid retention); seizures; decreased hearing or ringing in the ears; yellowing of your skin or eyes (jaundice); or abdominal cramping, heartburn, or indigestion. Other, less serious side effects may be more likely to occur.Rapid swelling of face or around eyes, Chest tightness or trouble breathing, Unexplained fever or sore throat or fever ,Unusual bleeding or bruising, Yellowing of skin or eyes, ecreased amount of urine,Severe stomach pain or bloody vomit, Black, tarry or bloody stools, Drowsiness or dizziness, Ringing in ears, Headache, Nausea, stomach cramps, or mild heartburn, Swelling of feet or legs or weight gain , Constipation or diarrhea severe rash, hives, or itching.

Contraindications

All naproxen products are contraindicated in patients who have had allergic reactions to prescription as well as to over-the-counter products containing naproxen or naproxen sodium. It is also contraindicated in patients in whom aspirin or other nonsteroidal anti-inflammatory/ analgesics induce the syndrome of asthma, rhinitis and nasal polyps. Both types of reactions have the potential of being fatal. Severe anaphylactic-like reactions to naproxen have been reported in such patients.

All products containing naproxen or naproxen sodium are contraindicated in patients with active peptic ulceration or active gastrointestinal bleeding, patients with asthma and in patients with haemorrhagic diathesis.

Interaction

One should not use this medicine with aspirin (or products that may contain aspirin) or ibuprofen. Naproxen can cause stomach bleeding. Drinking alcohol can make this worse. If you have 3 or more drinks of alcohol every day, ask your doctor if you should use naproxen. One drink of alcohol is the same as 4 ounces of wine, 12 ounces of beer, or 1 ounce of hard liquor (gin, whiskey, and others).

Interactions with other Medical Products and other Forms of Interaction

- Concomitant administration of antacid or cholestyramine can delay the absorption of naproxen, but does not affect its extent. Concomitant administration of food can delay the absorption of naproxen, but does not affect its extent.

- Naproxen is highly bound to plasma albumin; it thus has a theoretical potential for interaction with other albumin-bound medicines such as coumarin-type anticoagulants, sulphonylureas, hydantoins, other NSAIDs and aspirin. Patients simultaneously receiving naproxen and a hydantoin, sulphonamide or sulphonylurea should be observed for adjustment of dose if required.

- No significant interactions have been observed in clinical studies with naproxen and coumarin-type anticoagulants, however caution is advised since interactions have been seen with other nonsteroidal agents of this class, the free fraction of warfarin may increase substantially in some subjects and naproxen interferes with platelet function.Caution is advised when probenecid is administered concurrently, since increases in naproxen plasma concentrations and increased half-life of naproxen have been reported with this combination.

- Caution is advised when methotrexate is administered concurrently, since naproxen and other prostaglandin synthesis-inhibiting medicines have been reported to reduce the clearance of methotrexate, and thus possibly enhance its toxicity.

- Naproxen can reduce the anti-hypertensive effect of beta blockers.

- As with other non-steroidal anti-inflammatory medicines, naproxen may inhibit the natriuretic effect of frusemide.Inhibition of renal lithium clearance leading to increases in plasma lithium concentrations has been reported.

- It is suggested that naproxen sodium therapy should be temporarily discontinued 48 hours before adrenal function tests are performed, because naproxen may artefactually interfere with some tests for 17-ketogenic steroids. Similarly, Synflex therapy may interfere with some urinary assays of 5-hydroxy indoleacetic acid (5HIAA).

- Naproxen decreases platelet aggregation and prolongs bleeding time. This effect should be kept in mind when bleeding times are determined.

Pregnancy

As with other medicines of this type, naproxen produces delay in parturition in animals and also affects the human foetal cardiovascular system (closure of ductus arteriosus). Therefore, naproxen should not be used during pregnancy unless clearly needed.

Labour and Delivery

Naproxen-containing products are not recommended in labour and delivery because, through its prostaglandin synthesis inhibitory effect, naproxen may adversely affect foetal circulation and inhibit uterine contractions, thus increasing the risk of uterine haemorrhage.

Nursing Mother

The naproxen anion has been found in the milk of lactating women at a concentration of approximately 1% of that found in plasma. Because of the possible adverse effects of prostaglandin-inhibiting medicines on neonates, use in nursing mothers is not recommended.

Special Sense : hearing disturbances, tinnitus, visual disturbances.

Cardiovascular : dyspnoea, oedema, palpitations.

General : thirst.

The following adverse events have also been reported:

Gastrointestinal : abnormal liver function tests, colitis, oesophagitis, gastrointestinal bleeding and/or perforation, haematemesis, hepatitis (some cases of hepatitis have been fatal), jaundice, melena, nonpeptic gastrointestinal ulceration, pancreatitis, peptic ulceration, ulcerative stomatitis, vomiting.

Renal : haematuria, hyperkalaemia, interstitial nephritis, nephrotic syndrome, renal disease, renal failure, renal papillary necrosis, raised serum creatinine.

Haematological : agranulocytosis, aplastic anaemia, eosinophilia, haemolytic anaemia, leukopenia, thrombocytopenia.

Central Nervous System : aseptic meningitis, cognitive dysfunction, convulsions, depression, dream abnormalities, inability to concentrate, insomnia, malaise, myalgia, muscle weakness.

Dermatologic : alopecia, epidermal necrolysis, erythema multiforme, erythema nodosum, fixed drug eruption, lichen planus, pustular reaction, skin rashes, SLE (systemic lupus erythematosus), Stevens-Johnson syndrome, urticaria, photosensitivity reactions including rare cases resembling porphyria cutanea tarda ("pseudoporphyria") or epidermolysis bullosa. If skin fragility, blistering or other symptoms suggestive of pseudoporphyria occur, treatment should be discontinued and the patient monitored.

Special Senses : hearing impairment.

Cardiovascular : congestive heart failure, hypertension, pulmonary oedema, vasculitis.

Adverse Effect and Warnings

Like other NSAIDs, naproxen is capable of producing disturbances in the gastrointestinal tract. Taking the medication with food may help to alleviate this most commonly reported adverse effect. Also like other NSAIDs, naproxen can inhibit the excretion of sodium and lithium. Extreme care must be taken by those who use this drug along with lithium supplements. Naproxen is also not recommended for use with NSAIDs of the salicylate family (drugs may reduce each other's effects), nor with anticoagulants (may increase risk of bleeding).Certain preparations of Naproxen are not recommended for use in patients with hypertension, as they contain sodium, worsening the effects of hypertension.

In August 2006, the journal Birth Defects Research Part B published results in the September issue indicating that pregnant women who take NSAIDs including Naproxen in the first trimester run an increased risk of having a child with congenital birth defects, particularly heart anomalies.

Uses

Naproxen treats pain caused by arthritis, gout, menstrual cramps, and other medical problems. The over-the-counter brand is only for minor aches and pains and mild fevers. Belongs to a class of drug called non-steroidal anti-inflammatory drugs (NSAIDs).

Suprofen

History

Suprofen was originally introduced in U. S. in 1985 for the treatment of dysmenorrheal and as an analgesic for mild to moderate pain. Reports of sever flank pain and transient renal failure appeared abruptly within several hours after one or two doses and suprofen was removed from the U. S. market in 1987. Suprofen was reintroduced in the U. S. in 1990 as a 1% ophthalmic solution for the prevention of surgically induced miosis during cataract extraction.

Description

Suprofen is a white to off white powder odorless or having a slight odor, microcrystalline powder that is slightly soluble in water.

Chemistry

Suprofen is biosteric with ketoprofen in processing the para-thenoyl subsituent rather than the m-benzoyl of ketoprofen. In SAR of the suprofen molecule, thiophene is heterocycle and methyl as the a-alkyl subsituents on the acetic acid moiety was clearly optimal. The thiazole and pyrimidine derivatives were less active. Replacements of the carboxyl group by amide or anilide gave less potent compounds. Suprofen is approximately six times as potent as ketoprofen.

IUPAC name - a-methyl-4-(2-thienylcarbonyl)-benzeneacetic acid)

Molecular formula - $C_{14}H_{12}O_3S$

Chemical Structure

Pharmacodynamics

By inhibiting prostaglandin synthesis, suprofen reverses prostaglandin-induced vasodilation, leukocytosis, increased vascular permeability, and increased intraocular pressure. Also inhibits miosis, which occurs during cataract surgery. Suprofen binds to the cyclooxygenase-1 (COX-1) and cyclooxygenase-2 (COX-2) isoenzymes, preventing the synthesis of prostaglandins and reducing the inflammatory response. Cyclooxygenase catalyses the formation of prostaglandins and thromboxane from arachidonic acid (itself derived from the cellular phospholipid bilayer by phospholipase A_2). Prostaglandins act (among other things) as messenger molecules in the process of inflammation. The overall result is a reduction in pain and inflammation in the eyes and the prevention of pupil constriction during surgery. Normally trauma to the anterior segment of the eye (especially the iris) increases endogenous prostaglandin synthesis which leads to constriction of the iris sphincter.

Pharmacokinetics

Absorption : Suprofen is well absorbed orally .72% excreted in urine in 6 hr mainly as dihydrosuprofen glucuronide.

Distribution : Peak serum levels occurring within 1hr of oral administration

Metabolism and Elimination : Suprofen is extensively and rapidly metabolized to glucuronides of the unchanged suprofen, dihydrothiophene derivative, hydroxylated metabolite, and the terepthalic acid metabolite acking thiophene.

Dosage and Administration

Suprofen, brand named suprol, available as 200 mg capsules, has recommended dosages in adults of 200 mg every 4 to 6 hours as needed up to a maximum of 800 mg per day. It is also available in ophthalmic solution.

Clinical Efficacy

Clinical trials in patients with chronic pain due to osteoarthritis showed that a dose of suprofen, 200 mg 4 times a day, was equivalent in analgesic activity to aspirin, 650 mg 4 times a day, and to ibuprofen, 400 mg 4 times a day. In patients with dysmenorrheal, 200 mg of suprofen was equivalent to 400 mg of ibuprofen.

Therapeutic Uses

- Suprofen are used in the eye to lessen problems that can occur during or after some kinds of eye surgery.
- Sometimes, the pupil of the eye gets smaller during an operation. This makes it more difficult for the surgeon to reach some areas of the eye. Suprofen are used to help prevent this.
- Also, Suprofen are used after eye surgery, to relieve effects such as inflammation or edema (too much fluid in the eye).

Brand Name

In US - Ocufen, Profenal mu

In Canada - Indocid, Ocufen, Voltaren Ophtha

Other - Musterfen, Profenol, Srendam, Sulprotin, Supranol, Suprocil, Suprol, Topalgic.

Niflumic Acid

History

Niflumic acid was employed as an antipyretic – anti- rheumatic agent in 1935. The uricosuric properties of niflumic acid were noted before 1950, and it use continued through 1964, as late as 1967 it was used, for a long term treatment of gout.

Molecular Formula : $C_{13}H_9F_3N_2O_2$

IUPAC Name : IUPAC : 2-[[3-(trifluoromethyl)phenyl]amino]pyridine-3-carboxylic acid

Molecular Weight : 282.22.

Melting Point : 204°C.

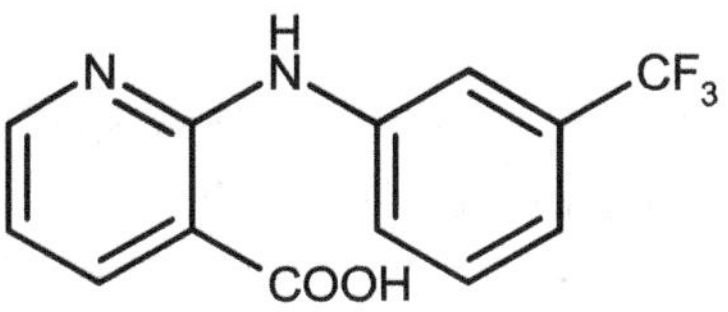

Pharmacodynamics

Niflumic acid is a nonsteroidal agent which has demonstrated anti-inflammatory, analgesic, and antipyretic activity in laboratory animals. The mode of action, like that of other nonsteroidal anti-inflammatory agents, is not known. Therapeutic action does not result from pituitary-adrenal stimulation.

In animal studies, Niflumic acid was found to inhibit prostaglandin synthesis and to compete for binding at the prostaglandin receptor site. *In vitro* Niflumic acid was found to be an inhibitor of human leukocyte 5-lipoxygenase activity. These properties may be responsible for the anti-inflammatory action of niflumic acid. There is no evidence that niflumic acid alters the course of the underlying disease.

Pharmacokinetics

Niflumic acid is reported to be well absorbed following oral administration, with measurable plasma levels being reached in 30 minutes and peak levels in 1-4 hours.

In studies on monkeys, highest Niflumic acid levels were detected in the plasma, liver, and kidneys. Lower levels were detected in skeletal muscle, fat, spleen, heart, and brain.

At plasma levels of 1 micrograms/ml, the drug was 99.8% bound to albumin. It rapidly crosses the placenta, but it is unknown whether it is distributed into milk.

The plasma half-life has been reported to range from 1-8 hours in horses. Therapeutic efficacy does not seem to be closely related with blood levels; however, as the onset of action may take 36-96 hours and significant efficacy may be seen for days following a dose.

Niflumic acid is metabolized in the liver primarily by oxidation to an active hydroxymethyl metabolite which may be further oxidized to an inactive metabolite (carboxyl). In humans, Niflumic acid and its metabolites are then excreted by the kidneys (approx. 70% within 7 days) or eliminated with the feces (20-30%). In horses, niflumic acid can be detected in the urine for at least 96 hours following the final dose.

Contraindication

The manufacturer states that Niflumic acid is contraindicated in animals with "active gastrointestinal, hepatic or renal diseases" Additionally; niflumic acid is contraindicated in patients demonstrating previous hypersensitivity reactions to it or salicylates. It is relatively contraindicated in patients with active or historical hemorrhagic disorders, or bronchospastic disease, because niflumic acid is highly bound to plasma.

Patients with hypoproteinemia may require lower dosages to prevent symptoms of toxicity. Niflumic acid has been shown to delay parturition in some species and therefore should be avoided during the last stages of pregnancy. It has caused teratogenic effects (minor skeletal abnormalities, delayed ossification) in rodents.

Drug Interation

Niflumic acid is highly bound to plasma proteins and may displace other highly bound drugs, increased serum levels and duration of actions of phenytoin, valproic acid, oral anticoagulants, and other anti-inflammatory agents. If niflumic acid is used concurrently with warfarin, enhanced hypoprothrombinemic effects may transpire.

When aspirin is used concurrently with niflumic acid, plasma levels of niflumic acid may decrease as well as a likelihood of increased GI adverse effects (blood loss) developing. Concomitant administration of aspirin with meclofenamic acid is not recommended.

Brand Name or Available As :

In India: Nifluril.

In Australia: Actol.

In Belgium: Niflugel.

In France: Flunir, niflugel, nifluril, gerj actol.

In Hong Kong: Nifluril.

In Italy: Niflam.

In Portgal: Nifloril.

In Spain: Niflactol.

In Swizerland: Niflugel, nifluril

Chapter 3

Enolic Acid Derivatives

History

After Second World War a German chemist Hans Stenzl synthesized phenylbutazone. 1,2 diphenyl – 4 – n – butylpyrazolidin 3, 5 – dion in the research laboratories of J. R. Weigy in Basel, Switzerland.

Description

Chemical name - 4-Butyl-1,2-diphenyl-3,5-pyrazolidinedione

Molecular formula – $C_{19} H_{20} N_2 O_2$

Molecular weight - 308.08

It is white or almost white, crystalline powder, practically odourles with a slightly bitter taste, soluble in 28 of ethanol, 1 in 1.25 of chloroform & 1 in 15 of ether, freely soluble in acetone, soluble in an alkaline solution and insoluble in water

Pharmacokinetics

Absorption

It is absorbed orally, 98% bound to plasma proteins and completely metabolized in the liver by hydroxylation and glucuronidation. The plasma t1/2 is 60 hours. It absorbed from GIT with peak plasma conc. occurring about 2 hours after ingestion. It also readily absorbed when administered, rectally. It is widely distributed throughout body fluids and tissue. It diffuses into the synovial fluid crosses the placenta & small accounts enter the CNS and breast milk. It is 98% bound to plasma proteins. It is extensively metabolized in the liver by oxidation & by conjugation with glucuronic acid. It is mainly excreted in urine as metabolites although about a quarter doses may be excreted in the faces. The plasma elimination half life is about two hours and it is subject to large inter-individual variation.

Drug Metabolism

Several authors have demonstrated that phenylbutazone underwent aromatic & side chain oxidation but the quantities in which the identified metabolites were present in human urine accounted for not more than a few percent of the dose. These amounts increased only insignificantly upon cleavage with B-glucronide unaltered it did not cover more than about 1% the elimination of the drug from blood is largely determined by biotransformations since only a very small amount is removed as unchanged phenyl-butazone by straight forward renal excretion.

Adverse Drug Reaction

1. Nausea, vomiting, epigastric distress, diarrhea, due to salt retention skin rashes, dizziness, drowsiness, headache, & blurred vision may, occur with phenylbutazone. More serious reactions include gastric irritation with ulceration, hepatitis, jaundice, haematuria, renal failure, and pancreatitis.

2. It may precipitate heart failure and may also cause an acute pulmonary syndrome with dyspnoea & fever.

3. Salivary gland enlargement hypersensitivity reactions including asthma & severe generalized reaction including lymphadenopathy, erythema multiforme, steverns-john son's syndrome toxic epidermal necrosis & exfoliative dermatitis have been reported.

4. The most serious effect of phenylbutazone are related to bone marrow depression & agranulocytosis & aplastic anemia.

5. Blood disorder may develop soon after starting treatment or may occur suddenly after prolonged treatment regular for their adverse effect on one blood of especially for total agronulocytosis & aplastic anaemia.

Adverse Effect

1. More toxic then aspirin.

2. Nausea, vomiting, epigastric destruct peptic ulceration are common.

3. Diarrhea of a variety of CNS side effect is reported.

4. Edema due to non retention is the major limitation of use for more then 1-2 weeks.

5. Hypersensitivity – Rashes, serum, sickness, Hepatitis of stomatitis.

6. Goiter of hypothyroidism have occurred on long term use.

Dosage and Administation

600 to 600 mg daily 100 to 400 mg daily.

Therapeutic Use

1. It is effective in all musucloskelatal and joint disorder including ankylosing spondylitis, acute gout, Osteoarthritis and rheumatoid arthritis.

2. It should only use acute condition where less toxic drugs have failed.

3. In UK use of phenylpulazone is restricted to the hospital treatment of ankylosing spondylitis unresponsive to other drug when the recommended initial dose is 200 mg given by mouth 2 or 3 times daily for 2 days. The dose in then reduced to the minimum effective amount which is usually 200 to 300 mg daily given in divided doses. Treatment should be given for the shortest periods possible. Elderly patients may require reduced dose.

4. In some countries phenylbutazone given as a rectal suppository and applied topically for musculoskeletal pain and in soft tissue injury.

5. It also given intramuscularly as the sodium salt.

6. Because of risk of fatal agranulocytosis & other serious reaction phenylbutazone have been banned in many countries with the availability of safer NSAIDs.

Oxyphenbutazone

History

History of non steroidal anti inflammatory drugs back to the nineteenth century. Oxyphenbutazone was employed as an antipyretic – antirheumatic agent in 1925. The uricosuric properties of oxyphenbutazone were noted before 1940 and its use continued through 1960, as late as 1965 it was used for a long term treatment of gout.

Description

A white crystalliine powder practically insoluble in water, freely soluble in alcohol, soluble in ether it dissolve in dilute solution of alkali hydrixide protect from light.

Chemistry

Many modification of the oxyphenbutazone structure have been made in the attempt to increase activity and reduce toxicity. There is a close relationship between the acidity and biological activity of the oxyphenbutazone derivatives. Increasing the acidity decreasing the anti-inflammatory activity and sodium-retaining potency but greatly increase the uricosric effect.

Molecular Weight - 324.38 (anhydrous), 342.39 (monohydrate).

It is white crystalline powder, odorless or almost odorless with bitter taste.

Pharmacodynamics

Oxyphenbutazone is a nonsteroidal agent which has demonstrated anti-inflammatory, analgesic, and antipyretic activity in laboratory animals. The mode of action, like that of other nonsteroidal anti-inflammatory agents, is not known. Therapeutic action does not result from pituitary-adrenal stimulation. In animal studies, oxyphenbutazone was found to inhibit prostaglandin synthesis and to compete for binding at the prostaglandin receptor site. *In vitro* oxyphenbutazone was found to be an inhibitor of human leukocyte 5-lipoxygenase activity. These properties may be responsible for the anti-inflammatory action of oxyphenbutazone there is no evidence that oxyphenbutazone alters the course of the underlying disease.

In several human isotope studies, oxyphenbutazone, at a dosage of 300 mg/day, produced a fecal blood loss of 1 to 2 mL per day, and 2 to 3 mL per day at 400 mg/day. Aspirin, at a dosage of 3.6 g/day, caused a fecal blood loss of 6 mL per day.

In a multiple-dose, one-week study in normal human volunteers, oxyphenbutazone had little or no effect on collagen-induced platelet aggregation, platelet count, or bleeding time. In comparison, aspirin suppressed collagen-induced platelet aggregation and increased bleeding time. The concomitant administration of antacids (aluminum and magnesium hydroxides) does not interfere with absorption of oxyphenbutazone.

Pharmacokinetics

Oxyphenbutazone is reported to be well absorbed following oral administration, with measurable plasma levels being reached in 30 minutes and peak levels in 1-4 hours.

In studies done with monkeys, highest oxyphenbutazone levels were detected in the plasma, liver, and kidneys. Lower levels were detected in skeletal muscle, fat, spleen, heart, and brain.

At plasma levels of 1 micrograms/ml, the drug was 99.8% bound to albumin. It rapidly crosses the placenta, but it is unknown whether it is distributed into milk.

Adverse Affect and Warnings

Adverse reactions are reported to be fairly uncommon in horses. However, hematologic changes (decreased hematocrit/PCV) and GI effects (buccal erosions, diarrhea, colic, anorexia, changes in stool consistency) have been reported. The diarrheal and colic reactions may be more likely in horses that have a heavy infestation of bots (*Gasterophilus* sp.) With chronic therapy, decreases in plasma protein concentrations may occur. In humans, NSAIDs have caused hepatotoxicity and it is recommended that human patients receiving chronic oxyphenbutazone therapy undergo occasional liver function tests. Although it does not appear that this adverse reaction is of major concern in either dogs or horses, the potential for hepatotoxicity does exist.

Drug Interaction

Oxyphenbutazone is highly bound to plasma proteins and may displace other highly bound drugs, increased serum levels and duration of actions of phenytoin, valproic acid, oral anticoagulants, other anti-inflammatory agents, salicylates, sulfonamides, and the sulfonylurea antidiabetic agents can occur. If oxyphenbutazone is used concurrently with warfarin, enhanced hypoprothrombinemic effects may transpire.

When aspirin is used concurrently with oxyphenbutazone, plasma levels of meclofenamic acid may decrease as well as a likelihood of increased GI adverse effects (blood loss) developing. Concomitant administration of aspirin with oxyphenbutazone is not recommended.

Uses and Indication

Oxyphenbutazone is used clinically in dogs for the symptomatic relief of symptoms associated with chronic inflammatory disease of the musculoskeletal system; often in an attempt to improve mobility in animals with hip dysplasia or chronic osteoarthritis.

In horses, it is indicated for the "oral treatment of acute or chronic inflammatory diseases involving the musculoskeletal system."

Pregnancy Category

In late pregnancy, as with other NSAIDs, NSAID should be avoided because it may cause premature closure of the ductus arteriosus.

Side Effect

Hypertension

NSAIDs can lead to onset of new hypertension or worsening of pre-existing hypertension, either of which may contribute to the increased incidence of CV events. Patients taking thiazides or loop diuretics may have impaired response to these therapies when taking NSAIDs. NSAIDs, including ANSAID, should be used with caution in patients with hypertension. Blood pressure (BP) should be monitored closely during the initiation of NSAID treatment and throughout the course of therapy.

Brand Name

Crovaril, Flogitolo, Flogoril, Frabel, Neo-Farmadol, Oxalid, tandacote, Tandearil, Tanderil, Visubutina.

Proprietary Name

In Australia : Tanderil.

In Brazil : Tandrez.

In Germany : Phloyonl.

In Mexico : butafen, edefen, maderil, oxabenol, fedolet, tandorene.

In Spain : Diflamin.

Routes of Administration : Oral

Piroxicam

History

Piroxicam was first developed by Pfizer and Co. about 15 years ago and in the seventies it entered into medicinal praxis. The pharmacological properties and therapeutic uses of piroxicam have been reviewed by Wiseman and by Lombardino.

Description

It is a white or slightly yellow crystalline powder. It shows polymorphism. It is practically insoluble in water, slightly soluble in dehydrated ethanol and aqueous alkaline solution, soluble in dichloromethane.

Systematic (IUPAC) name - 9-(hydroxy-pyridin-2-ylamino-methylidene) - 8-methyl-7, 7-dioxo-7$1^{6}$-thia-8-azabicyclo [4.4.0] deca-1, 3,5-trien-10-one.

Chemical Structure

Molecular Formula- $C_{15}H_{13}N_3O_4S$

Pharmacology

Piroxicam is in a class of drugs called nonsteroidal anti-inflammatory drugs (NSAIDs). Piroxicam works by reducing hormones that cause inflammation and pain in the body. Piroxicam is used to reduce the pain, inflammation, and stiffness caused by rheumatoid arthritis and osteoarthritis.

Pharmacodynamics

It is long acting NSAIDs with anti-inflammatory property similar to indomethacin and good analgesic-antipyretic action. It is a reversible inhibitor of COX, lowers PG concentration in synovial fluid and inhibits platelet aggregation – prolonging the bleeding time. Chemotaxis of leukocytes and ratio of T-helper to T-suppressor lymphocytes are reduced.

Pharmokinetics

Oxicam NSAIDs are a group of structurally closely related substances with anti-inflammatory, analgesic and antipyretic activities. They have a weakly acidic character and are extensively bound to plasma proteins. Piroxicam, the most widely used oxicam, is well absorbed after oral administration. Peak plasma concentrations (Cmax) of the drug are reached within 2 to 4 hours. Piroxicam has a small volume of distribution and a low plasma clearance. It undergoes hepatic metabolism and only 5 to 10% is excreted unchanged in urine. The elimination half-life varies between 30 and 70 hours. Age of the patient and renal or hepatic dysfunction do not seem to have any major effect on the pharmacokinetics of piroxicam. The drug reduces the renal excretion of lithium to a clinically significant extent, but the clinical significance of piroxicam-aspirin (acetylsalicylic-acid) and piroxicam-acenocoumarol interaction has not been established. Ampiroxicam, droxicam and pivoxicam are prodrugs of piroxicam that have been synthesized to reduce piroxicam-related gastrointestinal irritation. All prodrugs are well absorbed, but Cmax values are reached later than those following administration of piroxicam.

Absorption

Piroxicam is completely absorbed after oral administration, peak concentration in plasma occur within 2 to 4 hours. An antacid do not alter the rate or extent of absorption, but food may alter the rate.

Distribution

After absorption piroxicam is extensively (99%) bound to plasma protein. At steady state (e.g. after 7 to 12 days) concentration of piroxicam in plasma and synovial fluid are approximately equal.

Metabolism and Elimination

The major metabolic transformation in human being is cytochrome P450-mediated hydroxylation of the pyridyl ring (predominantly by an isozyme of the CYP2C subfamily) and this inactive metabolite and its glucoronide conjugate account for 60% of the drug excreted in the urine and faces. Less but than 5% of the drug   is excreted in the urine unchanged.

Adverse Drug Reaction

Common side effects are heartburn nausea and anorexia but it is better-tolerated and less ulcerogenic than indomethacin or phenylbutazone causes less faecal blood loss than aspirin. Rashes & pruritus are seen in less than 1% patients. Edema & reversible azotemia have been observed.

Digestive System : Anorexia, abdominal pain, constipation, diarrhea, dyspepsia, elevated liver enzymes, flatulence gross bleeding/perforation, heartburn, nausea, ulcers (gastric/duodenal), vomiting.

Hemic and Lymphatic System : Anemia increased bleeding time.

Nervous System : Dizziness, headache.

Skin and Appendages : Pruritus, rash.

Special Senses : Tinnitus.

Urogenital System : Abnormal renal function.

Body As Whole : Fever, infection, sepsis.

Drug Interactions

Aspirin : When piroxicam is administered with aspirin, its protein binding is reduced, although the clearance of free piroxicam is not altered. Plasma levels of piroxicam are depressed to approximately 80% of their normal values when FELDENE is administered (20 mg/day) in conjunction with aspirin (3900 mg/day). The clinical significance of this interaction is not known; however, as with other NSAIDs, concomitant administration of piroxicam and aspirin is not generally recommended because of the potential for increased adverse effects.

ACE-Inhibitors : Reports suggest that NSAIDs may diminish the antihypertensive effect of ACE- inhibitors. This interaction should be given consideration in patients taking NSAIDs concomitantly with ACE-inhibitors.

Diuretics : Clinical studies, as well as post marketing observations, have shown that piroxicam can reduce the rheumatic effect of furosamide and thiazides in some patients. During concoment therapy with NSAIDs, the patient should be observed closely for signs of renal failure.

Toxic Effect

The reported incidence of adverse effect in patients who take piroxicam is about 20% and approximately 5% of patient stop using the drug because of side effect. Gastrointestinal reaction are most common the incidence of peptic ulcer is less than 1%.Piroxicam and some other NSAIDs can reduce renal excretion of lithium to a clinically significant extant.

Dosage and Administration

Capsule, Suppositories, tablet gel, injection.

Therapeutic Uses

It is suitable for use sort term analgesic as well as long-term anti-inflammatory drug rheumatoid and osteoarthritis ankylosing spodylitis acute gout musculoskeletal injuries dentistry episiotomy dysmenorrhoea etc. Piroxicam approved in the U.S.A. for the treatment of rheumatoid arthritis and osteo-arthritis.

Brand Name

In India-Dolonex-10, 20mg capsule, 20mg dispersible tablet, 20mg/ml injection in 1 and 2 ml amps.

In America- Apo-piroxicam, Gen-pixicam.

In Canada – Pixicam, Buxicam.

Isoxicam

Description

Isoxicam is a nonsteroidal anti-inflammatory drug used to relieve the symptoms of arthritis primary dysmenorrhoea, pyrexia and as analgesics especially where there is an inflammatory component. It is also used in veterinary medicine to treat certain neoplasias expressing cyclooxygenase (COX) receptors, such as bladder, colon, and prostate cancers.

Chemical Name - 4-Hydroxy2methyl –N-(5Methyl-3-isoxazolyl)2H,1,2-benzothiazine-3-carboxamide 1,1,dioxide.

Molecular Formula- $C_{14}H_{13}N_3O_5S$

Pharmacodynamics

It is long acting NSAIDs anti-inflammatory property similar to indomethacin and good analgesic-antipyretic action. It is a reversible inhibitor of COX, lower PG concentration in synovial fluid and inhibits platelet aggregation – prolong the bleeding time. Chemotaxis of leukocytes and ratio of T-helper to T-suppressor lymphocytes are reduced.

Pharmacokinetics

Isoxicam was in widespread clinical use until its worldwide marketing was suspended because of fatal skin reactions. Isoxicam is completely absorbed, but Cmax values are not reached until 10 hours post dose. It has a low plasma clearance, approximately 5 ml/min (0.3 L/h), and low volume of distribution. The mean elimination half-life is 30 hours and does not appear to be affected by the age of the patient. Isoxicam potentiated the anticoagulant effect of warfarin, necessitating a 20% dosage reduction.

Absorption

Isoxicam is completely absorbed after oral administration, peak concentration in plasma occur within 2 to 4 hours. An antacid do not alter the rate or extent of absorption, but food may alter the rate.

Distribution

After absorption isoxicam is extensively (99%) bound to plasma protein. At steady state (e.g. after 7 to 12 days) concentration of isoxicam in plasma and synovial fluid are approximately equal.

Metabolism and Elimination

The major metabolic transformation in human being is cytochrome P450-mediated hydroxylation of the pyridyl ring (predominantly by an isozyme of the CYP2C subfamily) and this inactive metabolite and its glucoronide conjugate account for 60% of the drug excreted in the urine and faces. Less but than 5% of the drug is excreted in the urine unchanged.

Therapeutic Uses

It is suitable for use short term analgesic as well as long-term anti-inflammatory drug rheumatoid and osteoarthritis ankylosing spodylitis acute gout musculoskeletal injuries dentistry episiotomy dysmenorrhoea etc. Isoxicam approved in the U.S.A. for the treatment of rheumatoid arthritis and osteo-arthritis.

Adverse Drug Reaction

Common side effects are heartburn nausea and anorexia but it is better-tolerated and less ulcerogenic than indomethacin or phenylbutazone causes less faecal blood loss than aspirin. Rashes & pruritus are seen in less than 1% patients. Edema & reversible azotemia have been observed.

Toxic Effect

The reported incidence of adverse effect in-patient who takes Isoxicam is about 20% approximately 5% of patient stop using the drug because of side effect. Gastrointestinal reactions are most common the incidence of peptic ulcer is less than 1%. Isoxicam and some other NSAIDs can reduce renal excretion of lithium to a clinically significant extant.

Dosage and Administration

Capsule, Suppositories, tablet gel, injection.

Meloxicam

Description

Meloxicam is a nonsteroidal anti-inflammatory drug used to relieve the symptoms of arthritis, primary dysmenorrhea, and fever; and as an analgesic, especially where there is an inflammatory component. It is closely related to piroxicam.

Molecular Formula - $C_{14}H_{13}N_3O_4S_2$

Mol. weight - 351.403 g/mol

Systematic (IUPAC) name

(8E)-8-[hydroxy-[(5-methyl-1,3-thiazol-2-yl)amino] methylidene]-9-methyl-10,10-dioxo-10λ6-thia-9-azabicyclo[4.4.0]deca-1,3,5-trien-7-one

Approval Status

Meloxicam is quite popular in Europe for treatment of rheumatoid arthritis. It has recently (as of 2004) been approved for use in treating osteoarthritis in the United States.

The approval of meloxicam was the result of a "cluster" review approach, one of the process improvements FDA has instituted to facilitate the review of generic drug applications. FDA's Office of Generic Drugs (OGD) has begun to review groups of applications submitted at the end of 5 year new chemical entity (NCE) exclusivity in "clusters" to increase efficiency and decrease review time. At the expiration of 5 year exclusivity, FDA often receives multiple applications from different sponsors, submitted on the same day. In the case of meloxicam, OGD received over 20 abbreviated new drug applications (ANDAs) and FDA's review team effort resulted in the approval of 13 generic applications for this product in a little over 9 months of review time, resulting in the first time any generic version of this product is available.

Pharmacodynamics

Meloxicam is an NSAID and belongs to the class of drugs called enolic acid group, structurally related to piroxicam. Meloxicam significantly decreased symptoms of pain, function, and stiffness in patients, with a low incidence of gastrointestinal side effects. In models, it exhibits anti-inflammatory, analgesic, and antipyretic activities. Its mechanism of action may be related to prostaglandin synthetase (cyclooxygenase) (COX) inhibition.

Meloxicam has been shown, especially at its low therapeutic dose, to selectively inhibit COX-2 over COX-1.

Pharmacokinetics

Protein binding - 99.4%

Bioavailability - Not Known

Metabolism - Not Known

Half life 15 to 20 hours

Excretion - Not Known

Route/Dosage

7.5 to 15 mg once daily (maximum 15 mg/day).

Instructions For Use

Meloxicam comes as a tablet and suspension (liquid) to take by mouth. It is usually taken once a day with or without food.

Contraindications

Hypersensitivity to aspirin or any other NSAID.

Interactions

***ACE inhibitors (eg, captopril)* :** Antihypertensive effects may be decreased.

***Aspirin* :** Additive GI toxicity. Cholestyramine: Plasma levels of meloxicam may be reduced.

Loop diuretics (eg, furosemide), thiazide diuretics (eg, chlorothiazide): Diuretic effects may be decreased.

***Lithium* :** May increase lithium levels.

***Warfarin* :** May increase risk of gastric erosion and bleeding.

Lab Test Interferences: None well documented.

Adverse Reactions

CV : Arrhythmia; palpitation; tachycardia. DERM: Rash; pruritus; alopecia; angioedema; bullous eruption; erythema multiforme; photosensitivity;

Stevens-Johnson syndrome; sweating; toxic epidermal necrolysis; urticaria. EENT: Pharyngitis; esophagitis; abnormal vision; conjunctivitis; taste perversion; innitus. GI: Abdominal pain; diarrhea; nausea; constipation; dyspepsia; flatulence; omiting; colitis; dry mouth; duodenal ulcer; eructation; gastric ulcer; intestinal perforation; melena; pancreatitis; perforated duodenal and gastric ulcers; lcerative stomatitis. GU: Micturition frequency; urinary tract infection; albuminuria; increased BUN and creatinine; hematuria; interstitial nephritis; renal failure. HEMA: Anemia; agranulocytosis; leukopenia; purpura; thrombocytopenia; ilirubinemia. HEPA: Increased ALT and AST; hepatitis; jaundice; liver failure. META: Edema; dehydration. RESP: Upper respiratory tract infection; coughing; asthma; bronchospasm; yspnea. OTHER: Falling; flu-like symptoms; pain; arthralgia; back pain; anaphylactoid reactions.

Precautions

Pregnancy : Category C. Lactation : Undetermined. Children: Safety and efficacy not established. Elderly: Use with caution. Cardiovascular disease: Since fluid retention and edema can occur; use with caution in patients with fluid retention, hypertension, or heart failure. GI effects: Serious GI toxicity (eg, bleeding, ulceration, perforation) can occur at any time, with or without warning signs. Hepatic impairment: Assess liver function while on therapy. Renal impairment: Assess function before and during therapy because NSAID metabolites are eliminated by the kidney.

Indications

Meloxicam is used to relieve pain, tenderness, swelling, and stiffness caused by osteoarthritis (arthritis caused by a breakdown of the lining of the joints) and rheumatoid arthritis (arthritis caused by swelling of the lining of the joints). Meloxicam is also used to relieve the pain, tenderness, swelling, and stiffness caused by juvenile rheumatoid arthritis (a type of arthritis that affects children) in children 2 years of age and older. Meloxicam is in a class of medications called nonsteroidal anti-inflammatory medications (NSAIDs). It works by stopping the body's production of a substance that causes pain, fever, and inflammation.

Meloxicam is also used sometimes to treat ankylosing spondylitis (arthritis that mainly affects the spine). Talk to your doctor about the possible risks of using this medication for your condition.

Chapter 4

Non Acidic Compounds

Nabumetone

FDA Status

Nabumetone was approved by the Food and Drug Administration in December 1991.

Systematic (IUPAC) name

4-(6-Methoxy-2-naphthyl)-2-butanone

Mechanism of Action

It decreases inflammation, pain and fever, probably through inhibition of cyclooxygenase activity and prostaglandin synthesis.

Indications

Relief of symptoms of chronic and acute rheumatoid arthritis and osteoarthritis.

Contraindications

Hypersensitivity to aspirin, iodides or any NSAID.

Adverse Reactions

CV : Edema; weight gain; congestive heart failure; alterations in blood pressure; vasodilation; palpitations; tachycardia; chest pain; bradycardia. CNS: Dizziness; lightheadedness; drowsiness; confusion; increased sweating; vertigo; headaches; nervousness; migraine; anxiety; aggravated Parkinson's or epilepsy; paresthesia; peripheral neuropathy; myalgia; tremors; fatigue. DERM: Rash; urticaria; purpura. EENT: Blurred vision; tinnitus; rhinitis; salivation; glossitis; pharyngitis. GI: Diarrhea; ulceration; dry mouth; heartburn; dyspepsia; nausea; vomiting; anorexia; diarrhea; constipation; flatulence; indigestion; appetite changes; abdominal cramps; epigastric pain; hematemesis; peptic ulcer; stomatitis. GU: Acute renal insufficiency; interstitial nephritis; hyperkalemia; hyponatremia; papillary necrosis; melena; menometrorrhagia; impotence; menstrual disorders;

hematuria; cystitis; nocturia; proteinuria. HEPA: Hepatitis. HEMA: Increased prothrombin time; bleeding; anemia; neutropenia; leukopenia; pancytopenia; eosinophilia; thrombocytopenia. RESP: Bronchospasm; laryngeal edema; dyspnea; hemoptysis; shortness of breath. OTHER: Photosensitivity.

Precautions

Pregnancy : Category C. Lactation: Undetermined. Children : Safety and efficacy not established. Elderly patients: Increased risk of adverse reactions. GI effects : Serious GI toxicity (e.g., bleeding, ulceration, perforation) can occur at any time, with or without warning symptoms. Hypersensitivity: May occur; use drug with caution in aspirin-sensitive patients because of possible cross-sensitivity. Renal impairment: Lower doses may be necessary.

Tiaramide

History

Tiaramide history was seen on 12 June 1990.

Structure

Description

Tiaramide hydrochloride is a new non-steroidal anti-inflammatory agent previously shown to inhibit allergic responses both *in vitro* and *in vivo*. Clinical studies in asthmatic adults and children have also shown benefit.

Pharmacodynamics

It inhibits prostaglandin synthesis by decreasing the activity of the enzyme cyclooxygenase, which results in decreased formation of prostaglandin precursors.

Tiaramide inhibited the PGE2 release and contraction induced by bradykinin by reducing the arachidonic acid release from membrane phospholipid but did not have a direct effect on cyclo-oxygenase. Tiaramide reduced IP accumulation induced by bradykinin to an extent similar to indomethacin. However, tiaramide had no effect on IP accumulation induced by PGE2, although it potently inhibited the contraction induced by PGE2, which elicits contractions without affecting phospholipase A2. The rise in intracellular free Ca^{++} induced by PGE2 as well as bradykinin was inhibited by tiaramide.

Pharmacokinetics

Onset of action : 1 hour

Duration : 12-24 hours

Absorption : 90%

Metabolism : Hepatic; prodrug requiring metabolic activation to sulfide metabolite (active) for therapeutic effects and to sulfone metabolites (inactive)

Half-life elimination: Parent drug-7 hours; Active metabolite: 18 hours

Excretion : Urine (50%); feces (25%)

Drug Interactions

ACE inhibitors : Antihypertensive effects may be decreased by concurrent therapy with NSAIDs; monitor blood pressure.

Angiotensin II antagonists : Antihypertensive effects may be decreased by concurrent therapy with NSAIDs; monitor blood pressure.

Anticoagulants (warfarin, heparin, LMWHs) in combination with NSAIDs can cause increased risk of bleeding.

Other antiplatelet drugs (ticlopidine, clopidogrel, aspirin, abciximab, dipyridamole, eptifibatide, tirofiban) can cause an increased risk of bleeding.

Corticosteroids may increase the risk of GI ulceration; avoid concurrent use.

Cyclosporine : NSAIDs may increase serum creatinine, potassium, blood pressure, and cyclosporine levels; monitor cyclosporine levels and renal function carefully.

Hydralazine

Antihypertensive effect is decreased; avoid concurrent use. Lithium levels can be increased; avoid concurrent use if possible or monitor lithium levels and adjust dose. Sulindac may have the least effect. When NSAID is stopped, lithium will need adjustment again.

Loop diuretic efficacy (diuretic and antihypertensive effect) may be reduced.

Methotrexate

Severe bone marrow suppression, aplastic anemia, and GI toxicity have been reported with concomitant NSAID therapy. Avoid use during moderate or high-dose methotrexate (increased and prolonged methotrexate levels). NSAID use during low-dose treatment of rheumatoid arthritis has not been fully evaluated; extreme caution is warranted.

Ethanol/Nutrition/Herb Interactions

Ethanol : Enhance gastric mucosal irritation

Adverse Reactions : 1% to 10%:

Cardiovascular : Edema

Central nervous system : Dizziness, headache, nervousness

Dermatologic : Pruritus, rash

Gastrointestinal : GI pain, heartburn, nausea, vomiting, diarrhea, constipation, flatulence, anorexia, abdominal cramps.

Dosage

150-200 mg twice daily or 300-400 mg once daily not exceeds 400 mg/day.

Clinical Efficacy

Tiaramide hydrochloride is a new non-steroidal anti-inflammatory agent previously shown to inhibit allergic responses both *in vitro* and *in vivo*. Clinical studies in asthmatic adults and children have also shown benefit. We report a double blind cross-over study in 35 adult asthmatic patients comparing oral tiaramide 200 mg four times daily with oral salbutamol 4 mg four times daily and placebo. Symptoms and bronchodilator inhaler usage were recorded in diary cards and morning and evening peak expiratory flow rates were also monitored. Both tiaramide and salbutamol had a significant therapeutic effect compared with placebo. More patients preferred tiaramide to salbutamol and there were fewer side effects during treatment with tiaramide. Tiaramide may be a useful oral therapy in asthma particularly for those patients intolerant of oral beta-adrenergic agonists.

Therapeutic Uses

Treatment of Asthma

Inhibits the action of mediators released from mast cells and has direct smooth muscle relaxant properties. It may therefore have a beneficial effect in asthma. A double-blind crossover trial comparing the bronchodilator activity of tiaramide and placebo over 16 days was undertaken in 13 patients with asthma. Peak expiratory flow rate (PEFR) was recorded on three separate occasions every day and frequency of salbutamol aerosol usage was noted on a diary card. During treatment with tiaramide the mean mid-morning PEFR (362 1/min) was higher than mean PEFR on placebo (328) (P less than 0.001) as was the evening PEFR (378) compared with placebo (388) (P less than 0.001). There was a significant reduction in daily use of the salbutamol inhaler whilst on tiaramide compared with placebo Tiaramide may be a useful addition to existing prophylactic treatment for asthma.

Antiallergic Activity of Tiaramide

Tiaramide is an analgesic agent with antiallergic activity *in vivo*. We have investigated the antianaphylactic properties of tiaramide and its metabolites in three in vitro models of anaphylaxis; namely, IgE-induced release of histamine from rat mast cells and human basophils, and IgG1-induced release of histamine from guinea pig lung slices. Tiaramide and one of the metabolites, desethanol tiaramide (DETR), were found to inhibit immunologic release of histamine in all three of these in vitro models. Although tiaramide and DETR were less potent than disodium cromoglycate (DSCG) and/or proxicromil as inhibitors of mediator release, they were not cross-tachyphylactic to DSCG in the rat mast cell model. These data indicate that tiaramide is a unique inhibitor of histamine release whose mechanism of action differs from that of DSCG, and which in vivo is converted to a more potent metabolite.

Fluproquazone

Fluproquazone is a quinazolinone derivative with potent analgesic and antipyretic effects in addition to anti-inflammatory action. It has been shown to be effective in a variety of animal species after both oral and parenteral administration, and has duration of action of several hours. The compound is many times more potent than acetylsalicylic acid and clinically generally resembles ibuprofen and indoprofen in its pharmacological effects, but with the very important difference that, when given, to rats repeatedly over a period of days, it lacks significant ulcerogenic activity

A history of fluproquazone found in oral surgery in 1979.

IUPAC Name

4-(4-fluorophenyl)-7-methyl-1-(1-methylethyl)-2(1H)-quinazolin

Mechanisms of Action

Inhibition of Cyclooxygenase

Major mechanism of action of all available NSAIDs - mode of inhibition varies with each of the chemical categories.

Pharmacokinetics

Onset of action - 1 hour

Duration of action - 12-24 hours

Absorption - 90%

Metabolism - Hepatic; prodrug requiring metabolic activation to sulfide metabolite (active) for therapeutic effects and to sulfone metabolites (inactive)

Elimination Half-life

Parent drug : 7 hours

Active metabolite : 18 hours

Excretion

Urine (50%) feces (25%)

Drug Interactions

ACE inhibitors : Antihypertensive effects may be decreased by concurrent therapy with NSAIDs; monitor blood pressure.

Angiotensin II antagonists : Antihypertensive effects may be decreased by concurrent therapy with NSAIDs; monitor blood pressure. Anticoagulants (warfarin, heparin, LMWHs) in combination with NSAIDs can cause increased risk of bleeding. Other antiplatelet drugs (ticlopidine, clopidogrel, aspirin, abciximab, dipyridamole, eptifibatide, tirofiban) can cause an increased risk of bleeding. Corticosteroids may increase the risk of GI ulceration; avoid concurrent use.

Cyclosporine : NSAIDs may increase serum creatinine, potassium, blood pressure, and cyclosporine levels; monitor cyclosporine levels and renal function carefully. Hydralazine's antihypertensive effect is decreased; avoid concurrent use.

Lithium levels can be increased; avoid concurrent use if possible or monitor lithium levels and adjust dose. Sulindac may have the least effect. When NSAID is stopped, lithium will need adjustment again. Loop diuretic efficacy (diuretic and antihypertensive effect) may be reduced.

Methotrexate : Severe bone marrow suppression, aplastic anemia, and GI toxicity have been reported with concomitant NSAID therapy. Avoid use during moderate or high-dose methotrexate (increased and prolonged methotrexate levels). NSAID use during low-dose treatment of rheumatoid arthritis has not been fully evaluated; extreme caution is warranted. Thiazides antihypertensive effects are decreased; avoid concurrent use. Warfarin's INRs may be increased by piroxicam. Other NSAIDs may have the same effect depending on dose and duration. Monitor INR closely. Use the lowest dose of NSAIDs possible and for the briefest duration.

Ethanol : Avoid ethanol (may enhance gastric mucosal irritation).

Adverse Reactions

Cardiovascular : Edema.

Central nervous system : Dizziness, headache, nervousness.

Dermatologic : Pruritus, rash.

Gastrointestinal : GI pain, heartburn, nausea, vomiting, diarrhea, constipation, flatulence, anorexia, abdominal cramps.

Side Effects

The side effects of fluproquazone compared on rat gastric mucosal cyclic nucleotide phosphodiesterases (PDEs). Some of the drugs inhibited PDEs effectively, the Ki values being clearly lower than those of theophylline. Mostly the type of inhibition was apparently competitive. Acetylsalicylic acid and ibuprofen were ineffective. No unambiguous correlation between the inhibition of mucosal PDEs and clinically observed gastric irritation was found. However, the inhibition of PDEs may modulate gastric side-effects of NSAIDs.

Therapeutic Uses

Analgesic activity in patients with non-migrainous headache, Management of strains and sprains, Antipyretic activity and Oesteoporsis

Proquazone

History

The history of Proquazone found in 1982 in the treatment of juvenile rheumatoid arthritis.

Chemical Structure for Proquazone

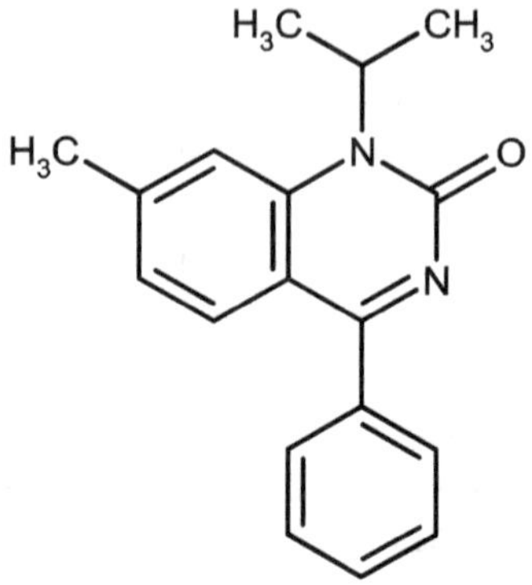

Pharmacokinetics and Pharmacodynamics

Absorption

Proquazone and its measured metabolites after intravenous administration show first order kinetics. The apparent half-lives of proquazone in plasma is 2, 14, and 76 min. The total clearance of proquazone is 700 mL/min, which indicates a high hepatic extraction.

Distribution

The apparent volume of distribution at steady state is 40 L, implying extensive binding or partitioning of the lipophilic drug in the tissues. Unchanged proquazone (<0.001%), the m-hydroxy metabolite (<1.0%), and the conjugated m-hydroxy metabolite (20%) are renally excreted after intravenous administration. The extent of absorption of proquazone is 7% and is entirely the result of a large first-pass effect.

Metabolism

A method for the determination of proquazone and its m-hydroxy metabolite in serum and urine by reversed-phase high-performance liquid chromatography is described. The technique is based on a single extraction of the unchanged drug, its metabolite and an internal standard from serum or urine with chloroform. The column was packed with mu Bondapak C18 and the mobile phase was acetonitrile--water (50:50) (pH 3). The detection limits for proquazone and its metabolite were 0.02 mumol/l using 500 microliters of sample. For the determination of the total m-hydroxy metabolite only 100 microliters of sample are needed. The method described is suitable for routine clinical and pharmacokinetic studies. The clinical application of this method suggests that the pharmacokinetics of proquazone in adults and children are similar.

Dosage

Proquazone of 75, 150, and 300 mg, a new nonsteroidal anti-inflammatory placebo in outpatients who had moderate or severe the relative potency of proquazone to aspirin ranged from to be dose related for proquazone.

Chapter 5

Miscellaneous

Celecoxib

Chemical Structure

IUPAC name

pyrazol-1-yl] benzenesulfonamide 4-[5-(4-methylphenyl)-3-(trifluoro-methyl)

Molecular formula - $C_{17}H_{14}N_3F_3O_2S$

Molecular Weight - 381.373 g/mol

Pharmacodynamics

Celecoxib is a highly selective COX-2 inhibitor and primarily inhibits this isoform of cyclooxygenase, whereas traditional NSAIDs inhibit both COX-1 and COX-2. Celecoxib is approximately 10-20 times more selective for COX-2 inhibition over COX-1. In theory, this specificity allows celecoxib and other COX-2 inhibitors to reduce inflammation (and pain) while minimizing gastrointestinal adverse drug reactions (e.g. stomach ulcers) that are common with non-selective NSAIDs. It also means that it has a reduced effect on platelet aggregation compared to traditional NSAIDs.

Pharmacokinetics

Celecoxib is absorbd from the GIT Peak plasma conc. being achieved after about three hours. Protein binding is approximately 97% celecoxib is

"

metabolized predominantly by the cytochrome P450 isoenzyme CYP2C9. Three identified metabolites are inactive as inhibitor of COX1 or COX2 enzymes it is eleminated mainly as metabolites in the faeces and urine less than 3% is recovered as unchanged drug. The effective terminal half-life is about 11 hour.

Adverse Effects

Aside from the incidence of gastric ulceration, celecoxib exhibits a similar adverse drug reaction (ADR) profile to other NSAIDs. Recently in a large study published in JAMA 2006, Celecoxib appears less adverse for renal (kidney) disease and heart arrhythmia compared to Vioxx.

Side Effects

Many recent studies have proven that Celebrex has many more side effects include stomach pain, constipation, diarrhea, gas, heartburn, nausea, vomiting, or dizziness. However there are another list of serious side effects that include heart attack, stroke, high blood pressure, heart failure from body swelling (fluid retention), kidney problems including kidney failure, bleeding and ulcers in the stomach and intestines, anemia (low red blood cells), life-threatening skin reactions, life-threatening allergic reactions, liver problems including liver failure, and asthma attacks in people who have asthma.

Brand Names

India-celebrax

U.S.A-celebra

Denmark-celebrax

Etoricoxib

Structure

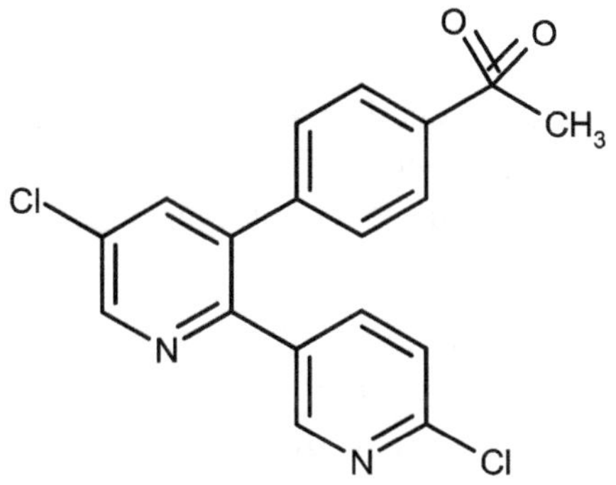

Chemical Structure

Etoricoxib is described chemically as 5-chloro-6'-methyl-3-[4-(methylsulfonyl) phenyl]-2, 3'-bipyridine. The empirical formula is $C_{18}H_{15}ClN_2O_2S$. The molecular weight is 358.84.

Physical and Chemical Properties

Appearance : Off-White Powder

Melting Point : 134-135°c

Pharmacodynamic

Etoricoxib exhibits anti-inflammatory, analgesic and antipyretic activities. Etoricoxib is a potent, orally active, selective cyclooxygenase-2 (COX-2) inhibitor. Two isoforms of cyclooxygenase (COX) have been identified: COX-1 and COX-2. COX-1 is responsible for prostaglandin mediated normal physiologic functions such as gastric cytoprotection and platelet aggregation. Inhibition of COX-1 by nonselective NSAIDs has been associated with gastric damage and platelet inhibition. COX-2 has been shown to be primarily responsible for the synthesis of prostanoid mediators of pain, inflammation and fever. Selective inhibition of COX-2 by Etoricoxib decreases these clinical signs and symptoms with decreased Gastro-intestinal toxicity and without effects on platelet function

Pharmacokinetics

Absorption

Orally administered etoricoxib is well absorbed. The mean oral bioavailability of etoricoxib is approximately 100%. The onset of action of etoricoxib occurs as early as 24 minutes after dosing. Following 120 mg once daily dosing to steady state, the peak plasma concentration (Cmax = 3.6 µg/mL) is observed at approximately 1 hour (Tmax) after administration to fasted adults & the AUC0-24hr is 37.8 µg•hr/mL.

Distribution

The volume of distribution at steady state is approximately 120 L in humans. Plasma protein binding of Etoricoxib is approximately 92% bound to human plasma protein over the range of concentrations of 0.05-5 µg/mL.

Metabolism

Etoricoxib is extensively metabolized. Metabolism of Etoricoxib is catalyzed by cytochrome P-450 enzymes. Five metabolites have been identified in man. These metabolites are only weakly active as COX-2 inhibitors.

Excretion

Elimination of Etoricoxib occurs almost exclusively through metabolism followed by renal excretion. The plasma clearance is estimated to be approximately 50 mL/min.

Indications

Etoricoxib is indicated in acute pain and inflammation, chronic musculo-skeletal pain, osteoarthritis, rheumatoid arthritis, acute gouty arthritis, primary dysmenorrhoea, ankylosing spondylitis.

Contraindications

Etoricoxib is contraindicated in the patients with known hypersensitivity to drug or to any of the excipients of this medicinal product, Active peptic ulceration or gastrointestinal bleeding, severe hepatic dysfunction, in Children and adolescents under 16 years of age and patients with inflammatory bowel disease and severe congestive heart failure.

Precautions

Etoricoxib should not be recommended to patients with decreased renal function and liver function, dehydration, hypertension, history of heart failure, perforation and people over 65 years of age.

Side Effects

Common side effects are dizziness, headache, gastro intestinal disorders (e.g., abdominal pain, flatulence and heartburn), diarrhoea, dyspepsia, nausea, asthenia, fatigue, flu-like symptoms. Rare side effects are edema, weight gain, anxiety, blurred vision, hypertension, epistaxis, dyspnoea, constipation, vomiting, muscle cramps, chest pain.

Drug Interactions

Rifampicin

Co-administration of Etoricoxib with rifampicin produced a 65% decrease in Etoricoxib plasma area under the curve (AUC).

Angiotensin Converting Enzyme (ACE) Inhibitors

Etoricoxib may diminish the anti hypertensive effect of ACE inhibitors.

Methotrexate

Etoricoxib may increase methotrexate plasma concentrations and reduce renal clearance of methotrexate when Etoricoxib at doses greater than 90 mg daily and methotrexate are administered concomitantly.

Aspirin

Concomitant administration of low-dose aspirin with Etoricoxib results in an increased rate of gastro intestinal ulceration or other complications compared to use of Etoricoxib alone.

Lithium

Etoricoxib may increase the plasma concentration of lithium.

Oral Contraceptives

Concomitant administration of Etoricoxib with an oral contraceptive containing ethinyl estradiol (EE) and norethindrone increases the steady state AUC0-24hr of EE.

Digoxin

Etoricoxib may increase the plasma concentration of digoxin.

Therapeutic Doses

Osteoarthritis : The recommended dose is 60 mg once daily.

Rheumatoid Arthritis : The recommended dose is 90 mg once daily.

Ankylosing Spondylitis : The recommended dose is 90 mg once daily

Acute Gouty Arthritis : The recommended dose is 120 mg once daily. Analgesia

Acute Pain : The recommended dose is 120 mg once daily.

Chronic Musculoskeletal Pain : The recommended dose is 60 mg once daily.

As the cardiovascular risks of selective COX-2 inhibitors may increase with dose and duration of exposure, the shortest duration possible and the lowest effective daily dose should be used. Patients on long-term treatment should be reviewed regularly, such as every three months, with regards to efficacy, risk factors and ongoing need for treatment.

Dosage and Administration

For adult and adolescent (over 16 years)

Arthritis, osteoarthritis : 60 mg once daily.

Rheumatoid arthritis : 90 mg once daily.

Acute gouty arthritis : 120 mg once daily.

Analgesia, Acute pain associated with dental surgery : 120 mg once daily

Brand Name

India-Arcoxia

U.S.A-Arcoxia

Nimesulide

History

It was launched in Italy for the first time as Aulin and Mesulid in 1985 and is presently available in more than 50 countries worldwide, among others France, Portugal, Greece, Switzerland, Belgium, Ireland, Mexico, and Brazil.

Description

Nimesulide is a prescription non-steroidal anti-inflammatory drug (NSAID) with analgesic and antipyretic properties and its approved indications are the treatment of acute pain, the symptomatic treatment of osteoarthrosis and primary dysmenorrhoea in adolescents and adults above 12 years old. Nimesulide is among the top 5 non-steroidal anti-inflammatory drugs worldwide.

Chemistry

IUPAC name - N-(4-Nitro-2-phenoxyphenyl) methanesulfonamide.

Molecular Formula - $C_{13}H_{12}N_2O_5S$

Mol Wt. - 308.311

Pharmacodynamics

Mechanism of action

The mechanism of action responsible for the effect seems to be inhibition of PGs synthesis by causing complete blockade of precursor enzymes cycloxegenase. Nimesulide is a sulphonilide compound .it is a COX2 inhibitor & devoid gastric toxicity. It also possesses such as inhibition of neutrophil activation and anti-oxidant property.

Pharmacokinetics

Absorption : Nimesulide is almost completely absorbed orally.

Distribution : It is 99% bound to plasma protein.

Metabolism : It is extensively metabolized in liver.

Excretion : Mainly by urine

Drug Interaction

Adverse drug reaction - Like most drugs in NSAID category, nimesulide is known to be hepatotoxic (damaging to the liver) in rare but unpredictable cases and should be taken with care. It did not achieve Food and Drug Administration (FDA) approval in the USA, and is banned in many countries due to cases of jaundice and hepatitis induced by its use. Italy was the first country to allow the drug in 1985. The European Medicine Evaluation Agency has prohibited the use of nimesulide for children under the age of 12.

Dosage and Administration

100 mg twice a day in osteoarthritis

Therapeutic uses - it is used as a pain inhibitor. Usually in case of arthritis.

Its probable mechanism is by acting on the COX receptors

Uses

It is used for short lasting pain full inflammatory conditions like sports injuries sinusitis and ear nose throat disorders, dental surgery dysmenorrhoea osteoarthritis.

Brand Names

India – Nise, Noble, Nimpac, Nimprex

Valdecoxib

Description

Valdecoxib is a prescription drug used in the treatment of osteoarthritis, rheumatoid arthritis, and painful menstruation and menstrual symptoms. It is classified as a nonsteroidal anti-inflammatory drug, or NSAID, and should not be taken by anyone allergic to these types of medications.

Valdecoxib was manufactured and marketed under the brand name Bextra by G. D. Searle & Company. It was available by prescription in tablet form until 2005, when it was removed from the market due to concerns about possible increased risk of heart attack and stroke.

Chemistry

IUPAC Name - 4-(5-methyl-3-phenylisoxazol-4-yl) benzenesulfonamide

Molecular Formula - $C_{16}H_{14}N_2O_3S$

Mol Weight - 314.364 g/mol

Pharmacodynamics

The mechanism of action responsible for the effect seems to be inhibition of PGs synthesis by causing complete blockade of precursor enzymes cyclogenase there are two iso-enzymes recognized for two cyclooxigenase COX1 & COX2. It is a selective COX2 inhibitor has no deleterious effect on stomach .it dose not inhibit COX1 and also dose not alters. Platelet function .it has anti inflammatory antipyretics and analgesic properties

Pharmacokinetics

Absorption - it is almost completely absorbed orally.

Distribution - It is 98% bound to plasma protein.

Metabolism - It is extensively metabolized in liver.

Excretion - Mainly by renal

Dosage and Administration

90 mg twice a day for reliving pain

Therapeutic Uses

Valdecoxib is used for musculoskeletal complaints, especially arthritis (rheumatoid arthritis, osteoarthritis, spondylitis, arthritis, ankylosing spondylitis), gout attacks, and pain management in case of kidney stones and gallstones. An additional indication is the treatment of acute migraines. It is used commonly to treat mild to moderate post-operative or post-traumatic pain, particular when inflammation is also present, and is effective against menstrual pain.

As long-term use of Valdecoxib and similar NSAIDs predisposes for peptic ulcer, many patients at risk for this complication are prescribed a combination of diclofenac and misoprostol, a synthetic prostaglandin analogue, to protect the gastric mucosa.

An external, gel-based form of Valdecoxib is available for the treatment of facial actinic keratosis which is caused by over-exposure to sunlight. Some countries have also approved the external use of Over-the-counter use against minor aches and pains and fever associated with common infections is also licensed in some countries.

In many countries eye-drops are sold to treat acute and chronic non-bacterial inflammations of the anterior part of the eyes (e.g. postoperative states).

Brand Names

India - Eject 90, BEXTRA

Chapter 6

Tabular Information

Table information of aspirin.

Pharmacological classification	NSAIDs
Therapeutic classification	Analgesic and anti-inflammatory.
Action	COX-2 inhibitor(non selective)
Empirical formula	$C_9H_8O_4$
Molecular weight	180.16
Melting point	148 - 149 C
Bioavaibility	55%
Metabolism	In liver
Elimination half-life	24 Hrs.
Excretion	By urine
Pregnancy category	Allowed
Routes of administration	Oral
Side effects	Nausea , vomiting
Available as	Oral solutions & tablets

Table information of diflunisal.

Pharmacological classification	NSAIDs
Therapeutic classification	Analgesic and anti-inflammatory.
Action	COX-2 inhibitor(non selective)
Empirical formula	$C_{13}H_8F_2O_3$
Molecular weight	250.20
Melting point	211-213 C
Bioavaibility	100%
Metabolism	conjugation with glucuronic acid
Elimination half-life	5 hrs.
Excretion	Through urine
Pregnancy category	Allowed
Routes of administration	Oral
Side effects	Nausea , vomiting
Available as	Oral solutions & tablets

Table information of benorylate.

Pharmacological classification	NSAIDs
Therapeutic classification	Analgesic and anti-inflammatory.
Action	COX-2 inhibitor(non selective)
Empirical formula	$C_{17}H_3NO_5$
Molecular weight	313.3
Melting point	178-181 C
Side effects	Nausea ,vomiting
Available as	Oral solutions & tablets

Table information of salsalate.

Pharmacological classification	NSAIDs
Therapeutic classification	Analgesic and anti-inflammatory.
Action	COX-2 inhibitor(selective)
Empirical formula	$C_{14}H_{10}O_5$
Molecular weight	258.2
Melting point	148-149 $^{\circ}$ C
Bioavaibility	90%
Metabolism	By Glucouronide complex
Elimination half-life	1.1 HR
Excretion	<1%,by urine in unchanged form
Pregnancy category	Not to be used
Routes of administration	oral
Side effects	Allergic reaction: Itching or hives
Available as	Tablets & capsules

Table information of sodium salsalate.

Pharmacological classification	NSAID Non narcotic analgesics
Therapeutic classification	Analgesic and anti-inflammatory.
Action	COX-2 inhibitor(selective)
Empirical formula	HOC_6H_4COONa
Molecular weight	160.10
Melting point	200 c
Pregnancy category	Allowed when emergency
Routes of administration	oral
Side effects	Nausea, dizziness, vomiting
Available as	Tablets & Enteric coated Tablets

Table information of trisalicylate.

Therapeutic classification	Analgesic and anti-inflammatory.
Action	COX-2 inhibitor (selective)
Empirical formula	$C_{26}H_{29}O_{10}NMg$
Molecular weight	539.8
Melting point	168 -169 C
Bioavaibility	99%
Metabolism	Through glucouronide complex
Elimination half-life	9 – 17 Hrs.
Excretion	Mainly Renal
Pregnancy category	Indicated when needed
Routes of administration	oral
Side effects	Indigestion, heartburn, diarrhea,
Available as	Oral solutions & tablets

Table information of diclofenac.

Pharmacological classification	NSAIDs
Therapeutic classification	Analgesic and anti-inflammatory.
Action	COX-2 inhibitor (selective)
Empirical formula	$C_{14}H_{11}Cl_2NO_2$
Molecular weight	296.148
Bioavaibility	100%
Metabolism	hepatic, no active metabolites exist
Elimination half-life	1.2-2 hr (35% of the drug enters enterohepatic recirculation)
Excretion	biliary, only 1% in urine
Pregnancy category	A(AU) B (1st. and 2nd. trimenon), X (third trimenon)
Routes of administration	oral, rectal, im, iv (renal- and gallstones), topical
Side effects	Indigestion, heartburn, diarrhea,

Table information of tolmetin.

Pharmacological classification	NSAIDs
Therapeutic classification	Analgesic and anti-inflammatory.
Action	COX-2 inhibitor (non selective)
Empirical formula	$C_{15}H_{14}NNaO_3$, $2H_2O$
Molecular weight	315.3
Melting point	155-157 $^{\circ}C$
Bioavaibility	Not more than 1%
Metabolism	Tolmetin glucuronide complex
Elimination half-life	Biphasic 1 to 2 & 5 hours resp.
Excretion	Through Urine
Pregnancy category	Avoided
Routes of administration	Oral
Available as	Capsules & Tablets
Side effects	. heart attack kidney problems including kidney failure

Table information of Zomepirac

Pharmacological classification	NSAIDs
Therapeutic classification	analgesic and anti-inflammatory.
Empirical formula	$C_{15}H_{13}ClNNaO_3$
Molecular weight	313.56
Melting point	178-179^{0}C
Bioavaibility	1.5%
Metabolism	Glucuronide complex
Elimination half-life	4-5 hours
Excretion	Exclusively through Urine
Pregnancy category	Avoided
Routes of administration	Oral administration
Available as	Tablets
Side effects	Stomach pain,constipation,heartburn nausea, vomiting.

Table Information of carprofen

Pharmacological classification	NSAIDs
Therapeutic classification	analgesic and anti-inflammatory
Action	COX inhibitor (non selective)
Empirical formula	$C_{15}H_{12}Cl\ NO_2$
Molecular weight	273.72g/mol
Melting point	197 ^{o}C
Bioavaibility	Approx 90%
FDA status	approved
Elimination half-life	8 – 12 hour
excretion	urine
Pregnancy category	contraindicated
Routes of administration	oral
Side effects	<ul><li>dizziness or headache;</li><li>nausea, diarrhea, orconstipation;</li><li>depression;</li><li>fatigue or weakness;</li><li>dry mouth; or irregular menstrual periods</li></ul>

Table information of ketorolac.

Pharmacological classification	NASID
Therapeutic classification	Pyrrolo-pyrole derivatives
Action	Analgesic, anti-inflammatory
Empirical formula	$C_{15}H_{13}NO_3$
Molecular weight	376.4 g/ml
Melting point	160 to 161 degree
Bioavailability	81 to 100%
Metabolism	Metabolites are the acyl gluronide,
Elimination half life	$T_{1/2}$ - 5-7 hr
Excretion	It is excreted by urine
Pregnancy category	"C"
Routes of administration	Oral, parental
Side effects	Weight Gain, dizziness, headache
Available as	Tablet, injection
FDA status	Approved

Table information of tromethamine.

Pharmacological classification	NASID
Action-	Analgesic and anti-inflammatory
Empirical formula	$C_4H_{11}NO_3$
Molecular weight-	121g/ml
Melting point-	171-172°C
Bioavailability-	75 to 85% oral
Metabolism-	Its metabolized by stomuch stage
Elimination half life-	4 to 6h
Excretion-	Excreted in urine
Pregnancy category-	"C"
Routes of administration-	Orally, perantraly
Side effects-	Respiratory depression, headeche
Available as-	Tablet, injection
FDA status-	Approved

Table information of mefenamic acid.

Pharmacological classification	NSAID
Therapeutic classification	Anti-inflammatory.
Action	COX-2 inhibitor
Empirical formula	C15H15NO2
Molecular weight	241.31
Melting point	230-231c
Elimination half-life	2 Hrs
Routes of administration	Orally
Side effects	Blood in urine or vomit
Available as	Tablets & Powder

Table information of flufenamic acid.

Pharmacological classification	NSAID
Therapeutic classification	Analgesic and anti-inflammatory.
Action	COX-2 inhibitor (non selective)
Empirical formula	C14H10F3NO2
Molecular weight	281.23
Melting point	133.0-135.0 degrees C
Elimination half-life	6-7 hrs
Available as	Tablets & Enteric coated Tablets

Table Information of pirprofen.

Pharmacological classification	NSAID
Therapeutic classification	anti-inflammatory.
Action	COX-1 inhibitor
Empirical formula	C14-H14-Cl NO2
Elimination half-life	9 Hrs.
Side effects	acute pain states.
Available as	Tablets & Enteric coated Tablets
FDA status	Not available

Table Information of fenbufen.

Pharmacological classification	NSAID
Therapeutic classification	analgesic and anti-inflame
Action	COX inhibitor (non selective)
Empirical formula	$C_{16}H_{14}O_3$
Molecular weight	254.3
Melting point	186°C to 189°C
bioavaibility	Approx86%
FDA status	Approved
Elimination half-life	10 hours-12 hours
excretion	Urine

Table Contd...

Pharmacological classification	NSAID
Pregnancy category	Contraindicated
Routes of administration	Oral
Side effects	Lungs disorders, Visual disturbances, Indigestion (dyspepsia), Abnormal reaction of the skin to light, usually a rash (photosensitivity), Retention of water in the body tissues (fluid retention), resulting in swelling (edema), Dizziness, Kidney damage, Severe blistering skin reaction affecting the tissues of the eyes, mouth, throat and genitals.(Stevens-Johnson Syndrome), Liver disorders, Hypersensitivity reactions such as narrowing of the airways (bronchospasm), swelling of the lips, throat and tongue (angioedema) or severe skin reaction (toxic epidermal necrolysis), Ulceration or bleeding of the stomach or intestines.

Table Information of flurbiprofen.

Pharmacological classification	NSAID
Therapeutic classification	analgesic and anti-inflamatory
Action	COX inhibitor(non-selective)
Empirical formula	$C_{15}H_{13}FO_2$
Molecular weight	244.3 g/mol
Melting point	244.27 $^{\circ}$C
Bioavailability	Approx 96%
FDA status	approved
Elimination half-life	4.7 and 5.7 hours
Excretion	Urine
Pregnancy category	Contraindicated
Routes of administration	Oral

Table Contd...

Pharmacological classification	NSAID
Side effects	• heart attack • stroke • high blood pressure • heart failure from body swelling (fluid retention) • kidney problems including kidney failure • bleeding and ulcers in the stomach and intestine • low red blood cells (anemia) • life-threatening skin reactions • life-threatening allergic reactions • liver problems including liver failure • asthma attacks in people who have asthma • stomach pain • constipation • diarrhea • gas • heartburn • nausea • vomiting • dizziness

Table information of ketoprofen.

Pharmacological Classification	NSAIDs
Therapeutic Classification	Analgesic ant rheumatic
Action	Anti-inflammatory, analgesic and antipyretic
Empirical Formula	$C_{16}H_{14}O_3$
Molecular weight	254.3
Melting point	94-97degree c
Metabolism	In the liver
Elimination half-life	2 hours
Excretion	Urine
Pregnancy category	C
Route of administration	Oral.
Side-effects	Photodermitis,
Available as	Tablet.
FDA Status	Approved

Table information of oxaprozin.

Pharmacological Classification	NSAIDs
Therapeutic Classification	Analgesic ant rheumatic
Action	Anti-inflammatory, analgesic and antipyretic
Empirical Formula	$C_{18}H_{15}NO_3$
Molecular weight	293.32
Melting point	160.5—161.5
Bioavailability	NA
Metabolism	In the liver
Elimination half-life	40 – 60hours
Excretion	By the urine
Pregnancy category	C
Route of administration	Oral & Topical
Side-effects	Dyspepsia, Urticaria
Available as	Ophthalmic solution & Tablet
FDA Status	Approved

Table Information of naproxen.

Pharmacological Classification	NSAIDs
Therapeutic Classification	Analgesic antirheumatic
Action	Anti-inflammatory, analgesic and antipyretic
Empirical Formula	$C_{14}H_{14}O_3$
Molecular weight	230-259
Melting point	70^0C
Bioavailability	95%(Oral)
Protein binding	99%
Half-life	1.8-2 Hour
Route of administration	Oral

Table information of suprofen.

Pharmacological Classification	NSAIDs
Therapeutic Classification	Analgesic ant rheumatic
Action	Anti-inflammatory, analgesic and antipyretic
Empirical Formula	$C_{14}H_{12}O_3S$.
Molecular weight	260.31
Melting point	$124.3^{\circ}C$
Bioavailability	NA
Metabolism	In the liver
Excretion	Urine.
Pregnancy category	C
Route of administration	Topical, Oral
Side-effects	Flank pain, Hematuria.
Available as	Capsules, ophthalmic solution
FDA Status	Approved

Table information of piroxicam.

Pharmacological Classification	**NSAIDs**
Therapeutic Classification	Analgesic antirheumatic
Action	Anti-inflammatory, analgesic and antipyretic
Empirical Formula	$C_{15}H_{13}N_3O_4S$
Molecular weight	331.35
Melting point	$198-200^{\circ}C$
Bioavailability	N.A.
Metabolism	4-10%renal
Elimination half-life	7-12 days
Excretion	Urine
Pregnancy category	C, D if used in the third trimester or near delivery
Route of administration	Oral, parental, topical
Side-effects	Heart burn, nausea Edema
Available as	Capsule, Suppositories, tablet gel, injection.
FDA Status	Approved.

Table Information of Isoxicam.

Pharmacological Classification	NSAIDs
Therapeutic Classification	Analgesic ant rheumatic
Action	Anti-inflammatory, analgesic and antipyretic
Empirical Formula	C14H13N3O5S
Molecular weight	335.34
Melting point	198-200^{0}C
Bioavailability	N.A.
Metabolism	4-10%renal
Elimination half-life	7-12 days
Excretion	Urine
Pregnancy category	C, D if used in the third trimester or near delivery
Route of administration	Oral, perentral, topical
Side-effects	Heart burn, nausea Edema
Available as	Capsule, Suppositories, tablet gel, injection.
FDA Status	N.A.

Table Information of tiaramide.

Pharmacological classification	Non – steroidal anti-inflammentary agents
Therapeutic classification	Anti-inflammentary, Analgesic, Antipyretic
Action	Inhibition of prostaglandin synthesis
Empirical formula	$C_{15}H_{18}ClN_3O_3S$
Molecular weight	391.0524
Bioavailability	90%
Metabolism	Desethanol, N-acetic acid N-oxide, N-acetic acid
Elimination of half life	1.3 hr
Excretion	extracted in urine in the first 12 hr.
Pregnancy category	Contra-indicated
Routs of administration	Oral
Side effect	Nausea, vomiting,dizziness
Available	Tablet (300mg-500mg)
FDA Status	Analgesic

Table Information of fluproquazone.

Pharmacological classification	Nonsteriodal anti inflammatory agents
Therapeutic classification	anti-inflammatory analgesic
Action	Prostaglandin synthesis inhibitor
Empirical formula	C18H17FN2O
Molecular weight	296.37
Bioavailability	90%
Metabolism	Phenolic derivatives
Elimination half life	Parent drug : 7 hours; Active metabolite : 18 hours
Excretion	Excreted in the urine and feces.
Pregnancy category	Contraindication
Routes of administration	Oral
Side effect	The inhibition of PDEs may modulate gastric side-effects of NSAIDs.
Available as	Tablet (75 to 200 mg), 100 to 150 mg,
FDA status	Analgesic and antipyretic

Table Information of proquazone.

Pharmacological Classification	Anti-inflammatory agents, non-steroidal Cyclooxygenase inhibitors
Therapeutic Classification	Analgesics, Anti-inflammatory
Action	Anti-inflammatory
Empirical Formula	$C_{18}H_{18}N_2O$
Molecular Weight	278
Bioavailability	90%
Metabolism	m-hydroxy metabolite
Elimination half life	Active metabolite : 18 hours
Excretion	Serum or ureine
Pregnancy category	Contraindication
Routes of administration	oral and intravenous
Side effect	gastrointestinal symptoms such as diarrhoea
Available as	(300 and 900 mg *via* capsules)
FDA status	Analgesic

Bibliography

Aberg, J.A., Zackin, R.A., Brobst, S.W., Evans, S.R., Alston, B.L., Henry, W.K., et al., AIDS Clinical Trials Group Study 5087., AIDS Res Hum Retroviruses. 2005, 21(9), 757-67.

Acetylsalicylic acid. Jinno Laboratory, School of Materials Science, Toyohashi University of Technology (1996).

Akhmedkhanov, et al. (2002). Br J cancer 87 (11): 1337-8. PMID 12085255.

Akhund L, Quinet RJ, Ishaq S. Archives of Internal Medicine. 2003 Jan 13;163(1):114-5.

Alegria P, Lebre L, Chagas C. Annals of Internal Medicine. 2002 Jul 2;137(1):75.

Alper AB, Jr., Meleg-Smith S, Krane NK. American Journal of Kidney Diseases. 2002 Nov; 40(5):1086-90.

Andrade, S.E., Gurwitz, J.H. and Fish, L.S., Med. Care, 1999, 37, 424-30.

Antony, S.J., Scand. J. Infect. Dis., 2006, 38(4), 293-5.

Aw TJ, Haas SJ, Liew D, Krum H. Arch Intern Med. 2005;165:490–6.

Baron, et al. (2003). N Engl J Med 348 (10): 891-9. PMID 12621133.

Bensen W, Weaver A, Espinoza L, et al. Rheumatology 2002 41:1008–16.

Berger P, Dwyer D, Corallo CE. Pharmacotherapy. 2002 Sep; 22(9):1193-5.

Bernareggi, A., Clin. Pharmacokinet. 1998, 35(4), 247-74.

Berry, H., Fernandes, L., Bloom, B., Clark, R.J. and Hamilton, E.B.D., Current Medical Research and Opinion 1980, 7,121-126.

Bjarnason, I., Zanelli, G. and Smith, T., Lancet, 1987, 2, 711-4.

Blot, L., Marcelis, A., Devogelaer, J.P. and Manicourt, D.H., Br. J. Pharmacol., 2000, 131(7),1413-21.

Blower A, Brooks A, Fenn G, Hill A, Pearce M, Morant S. Aliment Pharm Ther. 1997(11):283-91.

Bolesta, E., Kowalczyk, A., Wierzbicki, A., Eppolito, C., Kaneko, Y., Takiguchi, M., et al., J. Immunol., 2006, 177(1),177-91.

Bombardier C, Laine L, Reicin A, et al. N Engl J Med 2000; 343:1520–1528.

Bombardier C, Laine L, Reicin A, Shapiro D, Burgos-Vargas R, Davis B, et al.. N Engl J Med 2000; 343(21):1520-8. PMID 11087881.

Bombardier, C, Laine, L, Reicin, A, et al. N Engl J Med 2000; 343:1520.

Bort, R., Ponsoda, X., Carrasco, E., Gomez-Lechon, M.J. and Castell, J.V., Drug Metab Dispos., 1996, 24(8), 834-41.

Bort, R., Ponsoda, X., Carrasco, E., Gomez-Lechon, M.J. and Castell, J.V., Drug Metab. Dispos., 1996, 24(9), 969-75.

Bort, R., Ponsoda, X., Carrasco, E., Gomez-Lechon, M.J. and Castell, J.V., Drug Metab. Dispos. 1996, 24(8), 834-41.

Bosetti, et al. (2003). Br J Cancer 88 (5): 672-74. PMID 12618872.

Bosetti, et al. (2006). Eur J Cancer Prev 15 (1): 43-5. PMID 16374228.

Bree, F., Nguyen, P., Urien, S., Albengres, E., Macciocchi, A. and Tillement, J.P., Drugs, 1993,46 (1),83-90.

Bresalier RS, Sandler RS, Quan H, Bolognese JA, Oxenius B, et al., N Engl J Med. 2005;352:1092–1102.

Budavari, S., The Merck Index, 12th edn., Merck & Co., White House Station, N.J., 1996, 6640.

Carbaza, A., Carbre, F. and Rotten. E., J. Clin. Pharmacol., 1996, 505-12.

Carlson, J., Notis, W.M. and Corris, E.S., N. Eng. J. Med., 1990, 323, 135.

Catella-Lawson F, Reilly MP, Kapoor SC, Cucchiara AJ, De- Marco S, et al. N Engl J Med 2001;345:1809–17.

Caughey, GE, Cleland, LG, Penglis, PS, et al. J Immunol 2001; 167:2831.

Cervera R, Balasch J. Lupus 2004; 13(9):683-7. PMID 15485103

Chambers, H.F., Turner, J., Schecter, G.F., Kawamura, M. and Hopewell, P.C., Antimicrob. Agents Chemother. 2005, 49(7), 2816-21.

Chan, et al. (2004). Ann Intern Med 140 (3): 157-66. PMID 14757613.

Chan, et al. (2005). JAMA 294 (8): 914-23. PMID 16118381.

Chandrasekharan NV, Dai H, Roos KL, Evanson NK, Tomsik J, Elton TS, Simmons DL. Proc Natl Acad Sci U S A 2002; 99:13926-31. PMID 12242329

Charwizi, I., Ovwa, A. and Zinkin, H., J. Rheumtol., 1985, 12, 188-9.

Chauret, N., Lloyd, D.K., Levorse, D. and Nicoll-Griffith, D.A., Pharm. Sci., 1995, 1, 59.

Chenevard R, Hurlimann D, Bechir M, Enseleit F, Spieker L, et al. Circulation. 2003; 107:405–9.

Cheng, Y, Austin, SC, Rocca, B, et al. Science 2002; 296:539.

Crofford LJ, Lipsky PE, Brooks P, Abramson SB, Simon LS, van de Putte LBA. Arthritis Rheum 2000;43::4–13.

Crofford LJ, Oates JC, McCune WI, et al. Arthritis Rheum 2000; 43: 1891–6.

Dargan PI, Wallace CI, Jones AL. (2002). Emerg Med J 19 (3): 206-9.

Davis, R. and Brogden, R.N., Drugs, 1994, 48(3), 431-54.

De Almeida, M.A., Gaspar, A.P., Carvalho, F.S., Nogueira, J.M. and Pinto, J.E., Allergy Asthma Proc., 1997, 18(5),313-8.

De Leval, X., Dogne, J.M. and Delarge, J., Proceedings of the European League Against Rheumatism (EULAR), 2001, Jun   13-16,

De Radigues, X., Diallo, K.I., Diallo, M., Ngwakum, P.A,, Maiga, H., Djimde, A., et al., Trans. R. Soc. Trop. Med. Hyg., 2006, 8.

Deeks JJ, Smith LA, Bradley MD. BMJ 2002; 325:619.

Dhikav, V., Drugs News and Views, 2001, 6 (1), 64-5.

Dhikav, V., Sindhu, S. and Anand, K.S., IACM, 2002, 3 (4), 332-8.

Ding, C., Inflammation., 2002, 26(3), 139-42.

Dingle, J.T., J. Rheumatol., 1999, 58(3), 125-9.

Doomra, R. and Gupta, S.K., Intern. J. Med. Toxicol., 2001, 4 (1), 1-4.

Drandarska, I., Kussovski, V., Nikolaeva, S. and Markova, N. Int. Immunopharmacol., 2005, 5(4), 795-803.

Dudley Hart, F. and Huskisson, E.C., Drug, 1984, 27, 232.

Edwards JE, McQuay HJ, Moore RA. Pain 2004; 111:286–96.

Ernst EJ, Egge JA. Pharmacotherapy. 2002 May;22(5):637-40.

Estevez, F., Amaro, G., Giusti, M., Lasalvia, L. and Havranek, H., Medicina, 1993, 53(4), 307-14.

Fallavena, P.R.B. and Schapoval, E.E.S., lnt. J. Pharm., 1997, 158, 109.

Farkouh, ME, Kirshner, H, Harrington, RA, et al. Lancet 2004; 364:675.

FDA Advisory Committee Briefing Document Celecoxib and Valdecoxib Cardiovascular Safety. January 12, 2005–06–28.

FDA Arthritis Advisory Committee Meeting February 8 2001 Gaithersburg MD.

Fendrick AM, Bandekar RR, Chernew ME, Scheiman JM. Arthritis Rheum 2002; 47:36–43.

FitzGerald GA, Patrono C. NEJM 2001; 345:433–42.

FitzGerald GA. Am J Cardiol. 1991; 68:11B-15B.

FitzGerald GA. Coxibs and cardiovascular disease. N Engl J Med 2004; 351:1709–11.

Friedman B, Orlet HK, Still JM, Law E. South Med J. 2002 Oct; 95(10):1213-4.

Fries JF, Miller SR, Spitz PW, Williams CA, Hubert HB, Bloch DA. Gastroenterology. 1989; 96(2 pt 2 suppl):647–55.

Fries JF, Murtagh KN, Bennett M, Zatarain E, Lingala B, Bruce B. Arthritis Rheum. 2004; 50:2433–40.

Furberg, CD, Psalty, BM, FitzGerald, GA. Circulation 2005; 111:249.

Gabriel SE, Jaakinnainen L, Bombardier C. Ann Intern Med 1991;115:787–796.

Gandini, R., Montalto, C., Castoldi, D., Monzani, V., Nava, M.L., Scaricabarozzi, I., et al., Farmaco.,1991,46(9),1071-9.

Garcia Rodriguez LA, Varas C, Patrono C. Epidemiology 2000;11:382–7.

Garcia-Rodriguez LA, Jick H. Lancet 1994;343:169–173.

Garg G and Mishra P. , Indian J. Pharm.Sci., 2005,67(4), 489-491.

Garg G and Mishra P., J. Indian Chem. Society, 2006; 83: 103-104.

Garg G and Mishra P., J. Indian Chem. Society, 2006; 83: 288-290.

Gaudreault P, Temple AR, Lovejoy FH Jr. (1982). Pediatrics 70 (4): 566-9.

Giannoukas, A.D., Baltoyiannis, G., Milonakis, M., Nastos, D., Papagikos, L., Kappas, A.M., et al. World J. Surg., 1996, 20(4), 501-5.

Gibson, G.R., Whatacre, E.B. and Ricotti, C.A., Arch. Intern. Med., 1992, 152, 632-5.

Giglio P. South Med J. 2003 Mar; 96(3):320-1.

Giruad, M.N., Sandujask, Felder. Alim. Pharmacol. Ther. 1997, 11, 899-906.

Gomez-Gaviro, M.V., Gonzalez-Alvaro, I., Dominguez-Jimenez, C., Peschon, J., Black, R.A., Sanchez-Madrid, F. and Diaz-Gonzalez, F., J. Biol. Chem., 2002, 277(41), 38212-21.

Gonzalez-Alvaro, I., Carmona, L., Diaz-Gonzalez, F., Gonzalez-Amaro, R., Mollinedo, F., Sanchez-Madrid. F., et al., J. Rheumatol., 1996, 23(4), 723-9.

Goodman, Gilman's; The pharmacological Basis of Therapeutics. 10th ed., Mc Graw-Hill Companies, 2001, 691.

Gotzsche P. Controlled Clinical Trials. 1989; 10:31-56.

Graham D.J., Campen D, Hui R, Spence M, Cheetham C, Levy G, et al. Lancet. 2005; 365:475–81.

Graham D.Y., Agrawal NM, Campbell DR, et al. Arch Intern. Med. 2002; 162:169–175.

Graham, D.Y., Agrawal, M. and Donald, R.C., Arch. Intern. Med., 2002, 162, 169-75.

Grau, S., Antonio, J.M., Ribes, E., Salvado, M., Garces, J.M. and Garau, J., Int. J. Antimicrob. Agents, 2006, 57-63.

Green GA. Understanding NSAIDS: from aspirin to COX-2. Clin Cornerstone 2002; 3:50-59.

Griffin MR, Piper JM, Daugherty JR, et al. Ann Intern Med 1991; 114:257–263.

Grob M, Pichler WJ, Wuthrich B. Anaphylaxis to celecoxib. Allergy. 2002 Mar; 57(3):264-5.

Gscheidel D, Daspet MK, Le Coz CJ, Lipsker D. Hautarzt. 2002 Jul; 53(7):488-91.

Ha, S.J., Jeon, B.Y., Youn, J.I., Kim, S.C., Cho, S.N. and Sung, Y.C., Gene Ther., 2005, 12(7), 634-8

Hamam, R.N., Noureddin, B., Salti, H.I., Haddad, R. and Khoury, J.M., Ophthalmology., 2006,113(6), 950-4

Hansch, C., Sammes, P.G. and Taylor, J.B., Comprehensive Medicinal Chemistry, Oxford, 1990, 6, 711.

Hansch, C., Sammes, P.G. and Taylor, J.B., Comprehensive Medicinal Chemistry, Oxford, 1990, 6, 711.

Hansen, A. and Jensen, T., Ugeskr Laeger., 1998, 160(40), 5772-6.

Hassan-Alin, M., Andersson, T., Niazi, M., Liljeblad, M., Persson. B.A. and Rohss K., Int. J. Clin. Pharmacol. Ther., 2006, 44(3), 119-27.

Hatano, K., Yokota, Y., Hanaki, H. and Sunakawa, K., Kansenshogaku Zasshi., 2006, 80(3), 243-50.

Hawkey C, Laine L, Simon T, Beaulieu A, Maldonado-Cocco J, Acevedo E, et al. Arthritis & Rheumatism. 2000; 43(2):370-7.

Hawkey Jeffrey, C.J. and Karrasch. A., N. Eng. J. Med., 1998, 338, 727-34.

Henao J, Hisamuddin I, Nzerue CM, Vasandani G, Hewan-Lowe K. American Journal of Kidney Diseases. 2002 Jun; 39(6):1313-7.

Hennekens CH, Dyken ML, Fuster V. The American Heart Association. Circulation 1997;96:2751-3.

Hernandez-Pando, R., Aguilar-Leon, D., Orozco, H., Serrano, A., Ahlem, C., Trauger, R., et al. J. Infect. Dis., 2005, 191(2), 299-306.

Hillman RJ, Prescott LF. (1985). Br Med J (Clin Res Ed) 291 (6507): 1472.

Hinz, B. and Brune, K., Curr. Opin. Rheumatol., 2004, 16(5), 628-33.

Hoyo-Vadillo, C., Escobar, Y., Escobar-Islas, E. and Venturelli, C.R., Proc. West. Pharmacol. Soc., 2003, 46,168-9.

Hunt RH, Harper S, Watson DJ, Yu C, Quan H, et al. Am J Gastroenterol 2003;98:1725-33.

Huskisson, E.C., Irani, M. and Murray, F., European Journal of Rheumatology and Inflammation, 2000, Issue 1, 101-07.

Hutagalung, R., Paiphun, L., Ashley, E.A., McGready, R., Brockman, A., Thwai, K.L., et al. Thailand. Malar. J., 2005, 4, 46.

Hwang, J., Bitarakwate, E., Pai, M., Reingold, A., Rosenthal, P.J., and Dorsey, G., Trop. Med. Int. Health., 2006, 11, 789-99.

Jaworowski, A., Maslin, C.L. and Wesselingh, S.L., Sex Health., 2004, 1(3), 161-74.

John Robert Vane (1971). Nature - New Biology 231 (25): 232-5.

Johns, K.R. and Littlejohn, G.O. J. Rheumatol., 1999, 26(10), 2110-3.

Johnson AG, Nguyen TV, Day RO. Ann Intern Med. 1994 Aug 15; 121:289-300.

Jordan KM, Edwards CJ, Arden NK. Rheumatology. 2002 Dec; 41(12):1453-5.

Jovanovic D, Kilibarda V, Todorovic V, Potrebic O. Vojnosanit Pregl., 2005 Dec; 62(12):887-93.

Juni P, Nartey L, Reichenbach S, Sterchi R, Dieppe PA, Egger M. Lancet. 2004; 364:2021-9.

Kimmel SE, Berlin JA, Reilly M, et al. Ann Intern Med 2005;142:157.

King, J.R., Nachman, S., Yogev, R., Hodge, J., Aldrovandi, G., Hughes, M.D., et al., Pediatr. Infect. Dis. J., 2005, 24(10), 880-5.

Kirshenbaum LA, Mathews SC, Sitar DS, Tenenbein M. (1990). Arch Intern Med 150 (6): 1281-3.

Kivitz AJ, Nayiager S, Schimansky T, Gimona A, Thurston HJ, Hawkey C. Aliment Pharmacol Ther. 2004; 19: 1189–98.

Konstam MA, Weir MR, Reicin A, et al. Circulation 2001;104:2280.

Kovarik, J.M., Kurki, P., Mueller, E., Guerret. M., Markert, E., Alten, R., et al. J. Rheumatol., 1996, 23(12), 2033-8.

Kul'chavenia, E.V., Khomiakov, V.T. and Zhukova, I.I., Urologiia. 2004, (4), 34-7.

Kurahur, K., Matuhot. and Iide, M. Am. J. Gastroenterol., 2001, 96, 473-80.

Lai KC, Lam SK, Chu KM, et al N Engl J Med 2002; 346:2033–2038.

Laine L, Connors LG, Reicin A, Hawkey CJ, Burgos-Vargas R, et al. Gastroenterology 2003;124: 288–92.

Laine L, Maller ES, Yu C, Quan H, Simon T. Gastroenterology. 2004 Aug;127(2):395-402.

Landewe, R.B., Boers, M., Verhoeven, A.C., Westhovens, R., van de Laar, M.A., Markusse, H.M., et al., Arthritis Rheum., 2002, 46, 347-56.

Landewe, R.B., Boers, M., Verhoeven, A.C., Westhovens, R., van de Laar, M.A., Markusse, H.M., et al. Arthritis Rheum., 2002, 46(2):347-56.

Langman MJS, Weil J, Wainwright P, et al. Lancet 1994; 343:1075–1078.

Laporte, J.R., Ibanez, L., Vidal, X., Vendrell, L. and Leone, R., Drug Saf., 2004, 27(6), 411-20.

Legrand, E., Expert Opin, Pharmacother, 2004, 5(6), 1347-57.

Letzel, H., Megard, Y., Lamarca, R., Raber, A. and Fortea, J., Eur. J. Obstet . Gynecol. Reprod. Biol., 2006, 810-13.

Letzel, H., Megard, Y., Lamarca, R., Raber, A. and Fortea, J., Eur. J. Obstet. Gynecol. Reprod. Biol., 2006, 1245-51.

Lipsky PE, Abramson SB, Breedveld FC, Brook P., Burmester R., et al. J Rheumatol 2000;27:1338–1340

Lipsky PE, Brooks P, Crofford LJ, DuBois R, Graham D, Simon LS, van de Putte LB, Abramson SB Arch Intern Med 2000;160: 913–20.

Lipsy, P.E., Am. J. Med, 2001, 110 (3A), 4S-5S.

Litalien, C. and Jacqz-Aigrain, E., Paediatr. Drugs., 2001, 3(11), 817-58.

Litovitz TL, Klein-Schwartz W, White S, Cobaugh DJ, Youniss J, Omslaer JC, Drab A, Benson BE (2001). Am J Emerg Med 19 (5): 337-95.

Llorente Melero, M.J., Tenias Burillo, J.M. and Zaragoza Marcet, A., Rev. Esp. Enferm. Dig., 2002, 94(1), 7-18.

Loren, Lain. Gastroenterology, 2003,124, 288-92.

Lujan, M., Gallego, M. and Rello, J., Intensive. Care Med., 2006, 10.

MacDonald TM, Wei L. Lancet. 2003; 361:573–4.

Mahajan, S.S., Kamath, V.R. and Ghatpande, S.S., Parasitology, 2005, 131(4), 459-66.

Mamdani M, Juurlink DN, Kopp A, Naglie G, Austin PC, Laupacis A. BMJ 2004; 328:1415–6.

Mamdani M, Rochon P, Juurlink DN, et al. Arch Intern Med 2003;163:481.

Mamdani, M, Juurlink, DN, Lee DS, et al. Lancet 2004; 363:1751.

Martensson, A., Stromberg, J., Sisowath, C., Msellem, M.I., Gil, J.P., Montgomery, S.M., et al. Clin. Infect. Dis., 2005, 41(8),1079-86

Martindale, The Complete Drug Reference, 32nd edn. The Pharmaceutical Press, London, 1999, 63.

Mashimo, H., M Wu, D.C., Podolasky, D.K. and Fishman, M.C., Science, 1995, 274, 262-5.

McIntosh, H.M. and Jones, K.L., Cochrane Database Syst, Rev., 2005, 19.

McQuaid KR, Laine L. (2006). "Am J Med 119 (8): 624-38. PMID 16887404.

Mehandru S, Smith RL, Sidhu GS, Cassai N, Aranda CP. Thorax. 2002 May; 57(5):465-7.

Menezes, et al. (2006). Cancer Causes Control 17 (3): 251-6.

Meredith TJ, Vale JA. (1986). Drugs 32 (Suppl 4): 117-205.

Micheal, M.W., Am. J. Med., 1998, 15 (5A), 44S-52S.

Miller, R.S., Wongsrichanalai, C., Buathong, N., McDaniel, P., Walsh, D.S., and Knirsch, C., Am. J. Trop. Med. Hyg., 2006, 74(3), 401-6.

Moore DE. Drug Safety 2002; 25:345-72.

Moore R, Phillips C. Journal of Medical Economics. 1999; 2:45-55.

Morris, A.J., Madhock, R. and Stturock, R.D., Lancet, 1991, 337, 520.

Motaouakkil, S., Charra, B., Hachimi, A. and Benslama, A., Ann. Fr. Anesth. Reanim., 2006, 25(5),938-42.

Mottonen, T.T., Hannonen, P.J. and Boers, M. Clin. Exp. Rheumatol., 1999, 17(6 Suppl 18), S59-65

Mukherjee, D., Nissen, S.E., Topol, E.J., JAMA 2001; 286:954.

Nandakumar, D.N., Nagaraj, V.A., Vathsala, P.G., Rangarajan, P. and Padmanaban G., Antimicrob. Agents Chemother., 2006, 50(5):1859-60

Nduati, E.W. and Kamau, E.M., Acta Trop., 2006, 97(3), 357-63.

Ngondi, J.L., Oben, J., Etame, L.H., Forkah, D.M. and Mbanya, D., AIDS Res. Ther., 2006, 3(1),19

Nind G, Selby W. Intern Med J.2002 Dec;32(12):624-5.

Nussmeier NA, Whelton AA, Brown MT, Langford RM, Hoeft A, et al. N Engl J Med 2005;352: 1081–91.

Olive, G. and Rey,E., Drugs, 1993, 46 Suppl 1, 73-8.

Olofsson C.I., Legeby M.H., Nygårds F, Stman KM. Eur J Obstet Gynecol Reprod Biol 2000;88: 143–6.

Ostensen M.E., Skomsvoll JF. Expert Opin Pharmacother 2004;5(3):571-80.

Ott E, Nussmeier NA, Duke PC, et al. J Thorac Cardiovasc Surg 2003;125:1481 .

P.A. Insel, in Goodman & Gilman's The Pharmacological Basis of Therapeutics, 9 th edn., J.G. Hardman and L.E. Limbird, eds., McGraw Hill, New York, 1996, p. 644.

Palmieri, F., Cicalini, S., Froio, N., Rizzi, E.B., Goletti, D., Festa, A., et al., Int. J. STD AIDS., 2005, 16(7), 515-7.

Pandya, K.K., Satia, M.C., Modi, M.C., Modi, I.A., Modi, R.I., Chakravarthy, B.K., et al. J. Pharm. Pharmacol., 1997, 49, 773.

Parameters of the American College of Gastroenterology. Am J Gastroenterol 1998;93:2037–2046.

Pasero, G., Marcolongo, R., Serni, U., Parnham, M.J. and Ferrer, F., Curr. Med. Res. Opin., 1995,13(6), 305-15.

Pastorello, E.A., Zara, C., Riario-Sforza, G.G., Pravettoni, V. and Incorvaia, C., Allergy, 1998, 53(9),880-4.

Paternoster, D.M., Snijders, D., Manganelli, F., Torrisi, A. and Bracciante, R., Eur. J. Obstet. Gynecol. Reprod. Biol., 2003, 128.

Pathak A, Boveda S, Defaye P, Mansourati J, Mallaret M, Thebault L, et al. Annals of Pharmacotherapy. 2002 Jul-Aug;36(7-8):1290-1.

Perez Busquier, M., Calero, E., Rodriguez, M., Castellon Arce, P., Bermudez, A., Linares, L.F., et al. Clin. Rheumatol., 1997, 16(2), 154-9.

Peris, F., Martinez, E., Badia, X. and Brosa, M., Pharmacoeconomics., 2001, 19(7), 779-90.

Pertunnen K, Kalso E, Heinonen J, Salo J. IV diclofenac in post-thoracotomy pain. Br J Anaesth 1992;68:474–80.

Perucca E. Drugs., 1993;46 Suppl 1:79-82.

Pharmeuropa, Council of Europe, France, 1998, 10(4), 608.

Piel, B., Pirotte, I., Delneuville, P., Neven, G., Llabres, J., and Delattre, L., J. Pharma. Sci., 1997,86, 475.

Piyaphanee, W., Krudsood, S., Tangpukdee, N., Thanachartwet, W., Silachamroon, U., Phophak, N., et al. Am. J. Trop. Med. Hyg., 2006,74(3),432-5.

Ponsoda, X., Donato, M.T., Perez-Cataldo, G., Gomez-Lechon, M.J. and Castell, J.V., Altern. Lab. Anim., 2004, 32(2), 101-10.

Prieto de Paula, J.M., Romero Castro, R. and Villamandos Nicas, Y.V., Gastroenterol. Hepatol., 1997, 20(3),165.

Rabasseda, X., Drugs Today, 1997, 33, 41.

Rahal, J.J., Clin. Infect. Dis., 2006, 43 Suppl 2, S95-9.

Rahme E, Pilote L, LeLorier J. Arch Intern Med 2002; 162:1111.

Rainsford, K.D., Inflammopharmacology, 2006, 14(3-4), 120-37.

Rainsford, K.D., Rheumatology (Oxford), 1999, 38 Suppl 1, 4-10.

Rainsford, K.D., Rheumatology, 1999, 38, (1),4-10.

Raskin, J.B., Am. J. Med., 1999, 106 (S 5B), 3-12.

Ray WA, Stein CM, Hall K, et al. Lancet 2002; 359:118.

Reginster, J.Y., Paul, I. and Henrotin, Y., Rev. Med. Liege., 2001 56(7), 484-8.

Ridker PM, Cook NR, Lee IM, Gordon D, Gaziano JM, et al. N Engl J Med 2005; 352:1293–304.

Rossi S, editor. Australian Medicines Handbook 2006. Adelaide: Australian Medicines Handbook; 2006. ISBN 0-9757919-2-3

Sanchez, C., Mateus, M.M., and Henrotin, YE., J.Rheumatol., 2002, 29(4), 772-82.

Scharli, A.F., Brulhart, K. and Monti, T., J. Int. Med. Res., 1990, 18(4), 315-21.

Scheen, A.J., Rev. Med. Liege, 1999, 54(1), 62-4.

Schernhammer, et al. (2004). J Natl Cancer Inst 96 (1): 22-28. PMID 14709735.

Schneider F, Meziani F, Chartier C, Alt M, Jaeger A. Lancet. 2002 Mar 9; 359(9309):852-3.

Sekiguchi, Y., Yasui, K., Yamazaki, T., Agematsu, K., Kobayashi, N. and Koike, K., Clin. Infect. Dis., 2005, 41(11), 1158-63.

Sengupta, S., Velpandian, T., Kabir, S.R. and Gupta, S.K., Eur. J. Clin. Pharmacol., 1998, 54(7), 541-7.'

Sengupta, S., Velpandian, T., Sapra, P., Mathur, P. and Gupta, S.K., Pharmacology, 1998, 56(3),137-43.

Senol, G., Erbaycu, A. and Ozsoz, A., J. Chemother., 2005, 17(4), 380-4.

Shaya FT, Blume SW, Blanchette CM, et al. Arch Intern Med 2005;165: 181–6.

Shiraishi, Y., Kyobu, Geka. 2005, 58(8 Suppl), 724-8.

Sidhu, S., Kondal, A., Malhotra, S., Garg, S.K. and Pandhi, P., Indian J. Exp. Biol., 2004 42(12),1248-50.

Siegfried, N.L., Van Deventer, P.J., Mahomed, F.A., Rutherford, G.W. and Stavudine, Cochrane Database Syst. Rev., 2006, 19 (2), CD004535

Silva, C.L., Bonato, V.L., Coelho-Castelo, A.A., De Souza, A.O., Santos, S.A., Lima, K.M., et al. Gene Ther., 2005, 12(3), 281-7.

Silverstein FE, Faich G, Goldstein JL, et al. JAMA 2000; 284; 1247–1255.

Silverstein FE, Geis GS, Struthers BJ, et al. Gastroenterology 1994; 106(4):A180.

Silverstein, FE, Faich, G, Goldstein, JL, et al. JAMA 2000; 284:1247.

Simon LS, Smolen JS, Abramson SB, Appel G, Bombardier C, et al. J Rheumatol 2002; 29:1501–10.

Simon LS, Smolen JS, Abramson SB, et al. J Rheumatol 2002; 29:1501–1510.

Simon LS, Weaver AL, Graham DY, Kivitz AJ, Lipsky PE, et al. JAMA 1999; 282:1921–8.

Simon, L.S., Weaver, A. L. and Graham, D.Y., JAMA, 1999, 282 (20), 1921-8.

Simon, L.S., Weaver, A.L. and Graham, D.Y., JAMA, 1999, 282, 1921-8.

Singh G., Am. J. Med., 1998, 105 (1B), 31S-38S.

Singh, S., Sharda, N. and Mahajan, L., Int. J. Pharm., 1999, 176, 261.

Singla, A.K., Chawla, M. and Singh, A., J. Pharm. Pharmacol., 2000, 52(5),467-86.

Smith, M.B., Smith, R.H. and Jorgensen, W.L., Curr. Pharm. Des. 2006, 12(15), 1843-56.

Solomon DH, Glynn RJ, Levin R, Avorn J. Arch Intern Med 2002; 162:1099.

Solomon DH, Schneeweiss S, Glynn RJ, et al. Circulation 2004; 109:2068.

Solomon SD, McMurray JJV, Pfeffer MA, Wittes J, Fowler R, et al. N Engl J Med. 2005;352:1071–80.

Solomon, DH, Schneeweiss, S, Levin, R, Avorn, J. Hypertension 2004; 44:140.

Sowers, JR, White WB, Pitt B, Whelton A, Simon LS, et al., Arch Intern Med 2005;165:161–8.

Sowunmi, A., Fateye, B.A., Adedeji, A.A., Gbotosho, G.O., Happi, T.C., Bamgboye, A.E., Bolaji, O.M., et al., Acta Trop., 2006, 98(1), 6-14.

Stone, E (1763). Philosophical Transactions 53: 195-200.

Sun, H.Y., Fang, C.T., Wang, J.T., Kuo, P.H., Chen, Y.C. and Chang, S.C., J. Formos. Med. Assoc., 2006, 105(1), 86-9.

Tamblyn Robyn., Ann. Intern. Med., 1997, 127, 429-38.

Temple AR. (1981). Arch Intern Med 141 (3 Spec No): 364-9. PMID 7469627.

Thisted B, Krantz T, Stroom J, Sorensen MB. (1987). Acta Anaesthesiol Scand 31 (4): 312-6.

Thomas MC. Med J Aust 2000; 172:184-185.

Topol, EJ, Falk, GW. Lancet 2004; 364:639.

Topol, EJ. JAMA 2005;293:366.

Traversa G, Walker AM, Ippolito FM, Caffari B, Capurso L, Dezi A, et al. Epidemiology. 1995 Jan;6(1):49-54.

Tries, S., Neuper, T.W. and Laufer, S., Inflamm Res, 2002, 51 (3), 135-43.

Ugazio, A.G., Guarnaccia, S., Berardi, M. And Renzetti, I., Drugs, 1993,46 (1),215-8.

Vale JA, Kulig K; J Toxicol Clin Toxicol 42 (7): 933-43.

Van den Broek, I.V., Maung, U.A., Peters, A., Liem, L., Kamal, M., Rahman, M., et al. Trans. R. Soc. Trop. Med. Hyg., 2005, 99(10),727-35.

Van Steenbergen, W., Peeters, P., De Bondt, J., Staessen, D., Buscher, H., Laporta, T. and Roskams, T. J. Hepatol., 2000, 32(1), 174.

Van Tulder MW, Scholten R, Koes BW, Deyo RA. Non-steroidal anti-inflammatory drugs for low-back pain. Cochrane Database of Systematic Reviews. 2006(1).

Waddell, E.N. and Messeri, P.A., AIDS Behav., 2006, 10(3), 263-72.

Walson, P.D. and Mortensen, M.E., Clin Pharmacokinet., 1989,17 (1),116-37.

Ward, D.E., Veys, E.M., Bowdler, J.M. and Roma, J., Clin. Rheumatol., 1995, 14(6), 656-62.

Watson DJ, Rhodes T, Cai B, Guess HA. Arch Intern Med 2002;162:1105.

Weiss, R., Mitrou, P., Arasteh, K., Schuermann, D., Hentrich, M., Duehrsen, U., et al., Cancer, 2006, 106(7),1560-8.

Welte, T., Marre, R. and Suttorp, N., Med. Klin. (Munich)., 2006, 101(4), 313-20.

Whelton A, White WB, Bello AE, et al. Am J Cardiol 2002l; 90: 959–63.

Whelton, A, Fort, JG, Puma, JA, et al. Am J Ther 2001; 8:85.

White WB, Faich G, Borer JS, Makuch RW. Am J Cardiol 2003; 92:411.

White WB, Strand V, Toberts R, et al. Am J Ther 2004; 11:244–50.

Wilcox, C Mel., Arch. Intern. Med., 1994,154, 42-6.

Wilkes JM, Clark LE, Herrera JL. South Med J 2005; 98(11):1118-22.

Wolfe F, Zhao S, Pettitt D. J Rheumatol 2004; 31:1143.

Wolff, et al. (1998). Cancer Research 58 (22): 4997-5001.

Worret, W.I. and Fluhr, J.W., J. Dtsch. Dermatol. Ges., 2006, 4(4), 293-300.

www.answers.com

www.wikipedia.org

Yamazaki, R., Kawai, S., Mizushima, Y., Matsuzaki, T., Hashimoto, S. and Yokokura, T., Inflamm. Res., 2000, 49(3), 133-8.

Yang, C.C., Lee, M.H., Liu, J.W. and Leu, H.S. J. Microbiol. Immunol. Infect., 2005, 38(1), 47-52.

Yeka, A., Banek, K., Bakyaita, N., Staedke, S.G., Kamya, M.R., Talisuna, A., et al. PLoS Med., 2005, 2(7) 190.

Yeni, P., J. Hepatol., 2006, 44(1 Suppl), S100-3.

Yeoman, N.D., Am. J. Med., 2001, 110 (1A), 24S-28S.

Yeomans, Y.D., Tulassay, Z., and Juhász, L., N. Eng. J. Med., 1998, 338, 719-26.

Yong, C.S., Oh, Y.K., Lee, K.H., Park, S.M., Park, Y.J., Gil,Y.S., et al., Int J Pharm., 2005, 302(1-2), 78-83.

Zaragoza Marcet, A., Alfonso Moreno, V. and Roig Catala, E., Rev. Esp. Enferm. Dig., 1995, 87(6), 472-5.

Zawilla, N.H., Mohmmad, M.A.A., EL Kousay, N.M., and EL-Moghazy Aly, S.M., J.Pharm. Biomed. Anal., 2002, 27(1-2), 243-251.

Zongo, I., Dorsey, G., Rouamba, N., Dokomajilar, C., Lankoande, M., Ouedraogo, J.B., et al., Am. J. Trop. Med. Hyg., 2005, 73(5), 826-32

1. What are NSAIDs and how do they work?

2. For what conditions are NSAIDs used?

3. Are there any differences between NSAIDs?

4. What are the side effects of NSAIDs?

5. With which drugs do NSAIDs interact?

6. Give classification of NSAIDs according to heir half- lives.

7. "Do nonsteroidal anti-inflammatory drugs (NSAIDs) negate the antiplatelet effects of acetylsalicyclic acid (ASA)? What's the clinical significance?"

8. What are the symptoms of and treatment for a GI bleed?

9. Is there any serious health risks associated with diclofenac use?

10. What precautions should patient take before or while taking diclofenac?

11. What should patients tell healthcare professional before he or she prescribes Diclofenac?

12. What are the side effects associated with diclofenac?

13. Are there any interactions between diclofenac and other drugs or foods?

14. What should I do if I think I have been injured as a result of using diclofenac?

15. Are there Risks Associated valdecoxib Use?

16. Are there any Special Warnings with valdecoxib?

17. What general Precautions should require with valdecoxib?

18. What are some possible side effects of valdecoxib?

19. What is celecoxib used for?

20. Who should not take celecoxib?

21. What are the special warnings concerning the use of celecoxib?

22. What are the general precautions concerning the use of celecoxib?

23. What are some possible side effects of celecoxib?

24. What are the different uses for aspirin?

25. What is the basis for the aspirin prescribing information?

26. Is FDA concerned that some patients may self–treat?

27. If a consumer is interested in using aspirin to prevent or treat symptoms of heart problems, what should he or she do?

28. Do the data on treatment or prevention of cardiovascular effects pertain only to aspirin?

29. What should patients do if they are taking other pain medications such as ibuprofen?

30. What should consumers who are taking low dose aspirin for disease maintenance or prevention know about alcohol use?

31. Can consumers safely use aspirin to treat suspected acute heart attacks?

32. What do we know about how aspirin works for heart conditions and stroke?

33. Who should NOT take aspirin?

34. What other side effects are associated with aspirin?

35. What is key message for Consumers?

36. What were the major studies used to verify the effectiveness of aspirin for these indications?

37. What is the most important information we should know about diflunisal?

38. When are salicylates prescribed to treat arthritis?

39. Do salicylates carry the same cardiovascular risk as nonselective NSAIDs and COX-2 selective inhibitors?

40. Are other NSAIDs (e.g. ibuprofen, naproxen, COX-2 inhibitors) more commonly prescribed than salicylates?

41. Does Indomethacin cause the blood flow to increase or decrease to the brain?

42. Do we can take Indomethacin as a preventative or on onset of the migraine?

43. What are the side effects associated with Indomethacin?

44. What is the most important information I should know about ketorolac?

45. How does sulindac work in the body in cancerous cells, in normal cells?

46. What other uses does sullindac have?

47. What drugs are similar in function as sulindac?

48. What are the side effects of sulindac?

49. What is Rofecoxib?

50. What action did FDA take today?

51. What should I do if I am currently taking Rofecoxib?

52. What are the likely long-term health effects, if any, of taking Rofecoxib?

53. What other drugs are similar to Rofecoxib?